How to Make Yourself Exercise

How to Make Yourself Exercise

Exercise

Creating a Lasting Habit

By

James Rosen, Ph.D.

Sonoma, California

Library of Congress Cataloging-in-Publication Data

Rosen, James.
  How to make yourself exercise: creating a lasting habit / James
Rosen. – 1st ed.
  p. cm.
ISBN-13 9781548967741

Published by James Rosen, Ph.D. For further information, contact
howtomakeyourselfexercise@gmail.com

Back cover photograph: The author in his favorite outdoor office, by
Chas Blackford

Warning and Disclaimer
        In the interest of your safety, it is important to check with your
physician or medical care provider before beginning any exercise
program and to exercise according to your fitness level and
capabilities. Do not follow any suggestions in this book for type,
amount, or intensity of exercise unless you know or your physician or
medical care provider has told you that it is appropriate and safe for
your medical and physical condition.

Acknowledgements

My wife Julie has been with me through all my professional life in psychology. I often worked long hours. And for a good portion of our marriage I was a serious bicycle racer. During that time, for half of the year I traveled most weekends, leaving her alone with our young children more than she wanted. I gave up my car so I could commute to work by bicycle or running in order to get more workout time. That left her to drive the kids and do more of the errands. I appreciate that she supported me and managed to work around these and other inconveniences from my lifestyle. In addition to being my live-in psychology colleague and my occasional biking and hiking partner, Julie knew I had something unique to offer about this exercise problem and I appreciate how she nudged me to finish this book.

Were it not for my cycling and ski buddies I would not have had the inspiration to work out so consistently let alone to become an athlete. They've been great motivators to exercise. I can hardly do a bike ride now without other people to ride with. And importantly for this book, my friends have been a laboratory of wisdom and case studies for how to create a physically active lifestyle. That includes my friends' amateur psychology on everything from coping with the pain of hard workouts to coping with spouses who are not as gonzo about cycling or skiing.

Both my wife and friends tease me that it's taken so long to write this because I've been too busy exercising. They probably doubted that it would be finished, let alone published. Although they had reason to be skeptical, they humored me when I said, "I'm writing a book". To them and the people who said hurry and finish because they needed my advice on how to exercise more, thank you.

Finally, I want to thank my patients whom I admire for making exercise a bigger part of their lives. They truly have been the test lab and inspiration for this book. My patients taught me the tricks and excuses people make for not changing their health behavior. They taught me that an exercise habit is a psychological not just fitness challenge. They tolerated the technical and professorial way I presented information. And they used it to make huge increases in exercise and fitness. That gave me the confidence I could pull together all those talks and handouts into a single volume that hopefully other people will find as helpful as did they.

Table of Contents

Preface

As I was preparing to retire from psychology, I planned to write a book called "Losing Weight the Hard Way". Although there were many good weight loss books on the market, I thought most authors made it sound too easy to change eating and exercise and did not address the longer-term problem of creating habits that last. The "Hard Way" required self-control and sacrifice, not a quick and easy solution.

My friends and colleagues appreciated my point, but insisted the title would not sell books. Maybe lucky for me, I switched to writing this book, focused on the problem of creating an exercise habit. I did that because it turned out people who attended my lectures on weight control were more curious about how I taught my patients to exercise so much.

Sure enough, the psychology behind weight control programs focuses on eating less food rather than exercising more. There is a hole in the weight loss field and for that matter, in the health behavior field generally, that I decided to fill with a book focused on behavioral techniques to develop an exercise habit. It would be called, "How to Make Yourself Exercise" because for most people, exercise is not natural, it's something that you must force yourself to do, at least at the beginning. I wrote this book because it's about time the principles of self-control and learning are applied to one of the most difficult behaviors to incorporate into modern life. I wanted to present more than just tips on what to do, but the psychology, the science behind self-management. How to do it. Why it works.

I had many years of experience in weight control and taught over 500 participants in my program at the University of Vermont with some of the best results in the country. I know the information and homework in this volume help people to make big changes in their physical activity. I have the data on exercise change and weight loss to prove it. Moreover, if my approach works with seriously overweight adults with medical problems and little history of exercising, it should work with most anyone.

My approach to exercise also developed out of my clinical and research programs with physical injury and disability, eating disorders and body image disturbance, and anxiety and depression. People with these problems struggle with exercise as well and have concerns about fitness and physical self-image. During my career as a professor at the University of Vermont, I published over 100 scientific articles, chapters and books and taught courses on health psychology. This book is based on science, but I'm not presenting psychology from the armchair only. I'm writing from real personal experience.

As a young man I was into sports and physical recreation in a very casual and sporadic way. Then suddenly at age 35 I started bicycle racing and later cross-country ski racing. I won races and was a national champion. At age 68 I'm still a competitive athlete. I have experience with making myself exercise almost every day no matter what the weather or other responsibilities. I know all the excuses and mind games that interfere with exercising. And I know the self-talk, self-discipline and self-motivation needed to overcome them. I know how to apply the theory of developing a habit to real people with real obstacles.

James Rosen, Ph.D.

Professor Emeritus of Psychology

Sonoma, California

October 2017

Chapter 1:

Introduction

Why This Book Is For You

Like most people, you probably are not physically active enough to be truly healthy and happy. Sooner or later, something will happen that wakes you up or already has woken you up to the fact you need to do something about it.

Did your doctor warn you to exercise more? Is your family worried that you are not taking care of yourself? Maybe you feel frustrated that it's harder to do physical things. Are you not playing sports or exploring the outdoors with friends anymore? Or maybe you don't like your extra weight. You know you need to exercise more, but how to make yourself?

Usually people have to try several times before they finally change a health habit. What have you tried? Did you try to motivate yourself by joining a fitness center? Bought new exercise gear hoping you'd like to exercise? Did you try making a bet or a contest with someone? There are a lot of gimmicks and advice out there. But changing habits is not easy. How do you change and make it last?

Maybe you are already an expert in starting habit change. You have an activity that you enjoy. You have partners you can exercise with. You have the time to do it. And in the past you've had big improvements with just a short period of exercising. Yet, over and over, in weeks, months or even more than a year, your exercise habit disappears.

Maybe you have good explanations for quitting like your work hours changed, you are injured, or the weather is bad. Regardless, once you slip from your routine, to regain control feels like starting all over, maybe even harder than the last time. You want to have a lasting habit, but how not to slip, how to not backslide and lose your habit?

How about having some physical disability and being really limited? Feeling too much pain or even fear of exercising has made you give up. How do you overcome that?

Solving these exercise problems is the purpose of this book. You can learn how to gradually increase your physical activity and to make exercise a habit that lasts using techniques based on psychological principles of learning new behavior.

How This Book Is Different From Other Exercise Books

Unlike the typical how-to book on exercise, this one will not lecture on the health benefits of exercise. You probably know that exercise is really good for you and have even more reasons for becoming physically active. Nor will this book teach you specific types of exercise. You probably already know which exercise is good for you. If not, you can find good information on physical fitness and exercise in many other books, magazines, and websites.

But as far as I know, you will not find a book like this that is strictly focused on the psychology of "how to make yourself exercise". All the information on good ways to improve fitness is useless, unless you actually can make yourself get out the door to do it. That is my purpose; to make you get out the door and be more physically active. The goal is to make you an exerciser; to make you more physically fit is just the icing on the cake.

Certainly, there are many good suggestions for exercise motivation in the popular media such as: "Picture yourself in great shape. This will help inspire you." "Find an exercise buddy." "Pick an exercise you like." Do these sound familiar? Usually such tips are listed in a flashy magazine article or in a short chapter at the end of a weight control or fitness book. Maybe they will help, but in the end, not very much. That's because they are presented superficially without enough concrete instruction on how to implement them. More importantly, they do not address the bigger picture of how one creates a habit.

Instead, I will teach you a system of self-control that goes step-by-step beginning with techniques to make you just start exercising and then to more advanced strategies to make exercise a bigger part of your life. Along the way, you will learn the psychological principles underlying each technique that will help you to tailor it to your own situation. Unlike the superficial behavioral tips you can find elsewhere, I will teach habit techniques in-depth so you really will know how to use them.

Most authors try to inspire their readers with upbeat talk and positive affirmations about their ability to form an exercise habit. "Just two weeks to an exercise habit!" Do claims like this sound familiar? It's as if just saying something is easy should be enough to improve people's attitude. It is fine to be optimistic when setting out on a new exercise attempt, but to become a regular exerciser is not easy. You already know that it isn't. A habit takes way longer than two weeks. The light-hearted talk in most writings on exercise can backfire, because the readers give up when they discover they are not having the same happy, easy result as the image presented by the writer. My approach is to acknowledge the real difficulties people encounter when trying to create an exercise habit and to teach you how to deal with them.

Finally, most sources for people who need to exercise are too easy on the reader because they aim at very modest increases in physical activity, usually below what is truly needed for a major improvement in physical fitness and more importantly, for the creation of a strong habit. The hidden belief among authors, and national health organizations for that matter, is that if you present a goal too high above typical exercise levels, they'll feel overwhelmed and might give up. Therefore, the reasoning seems to be, it's better to give people an easier goal. They might feel more motivated and although, not ideal, they still will be healthier if they achieve it.

This book is focused on forming a habit and making exercise resistant to perishing. A large increase in exercise is needed for a strong habit. Hopefully, I will convince you that such a goal is achievable and the steps I give you will make it happen.

My Psychological Approach

My approach is not psychodynamic or psychoanalytic. Those psychologies might look to uncover some early experience to explain why a person avoids exercise. For instance, it could be that someone was teased playing sports as a youngster and now as an adult feels anxious about engaging in physical recreation. But given that the overwhelming majority of Americans do not exercise enough, the problem is too widespread to say it's a psychological condition that needs therapy.

My approach is called behavioral self-management. This involves concrete steps and skills to control and direct your behavior in order to achieve your objective of exercising more. It is based on behavior modification and cognitive behavior therapy, two related disciplines for changing behavior in people who either are well adjusted or have mental health problems. Two essential characteristics of behavioral self-management are 1) the techniques for change have been demonstrated by clinical science to be effective and 2) the objective is to change measureable behavior, not necessarily emotions or subjective states which are difficult to measure. Exercise is an ideal candidate for a behavioral approach because it is a behavior.

Using a behavioral approach does not mean I will ignore your feelings. I will help you look at emotions, thoughts and self-image that might be causing you to struggle with exercise. And although the bottom line is changing behavior, I will teach you how to manage these other influences in order to exercise more.

I will prescribe gradual changes in the amount, frequency, variety and circumstances of your exercise. As a behaviorist, I will dictate, but dictate humanistically, the changes that are required to form a habit. For the most part, I will not tell you what kind of exercise to do. I will encourage you to set your own goals and create challenges to grow as an exerciser. I will help you be more honest, aware and self-confident about your ability to exercise.

How To Use This Book

I assume you are ready to start exercising more. That means you think it's a good idea and you've thought through some of the pros and cons of starting right now. You've made a decision and you plan to change. Your mind is made up. This book is designed to translate that good intention into action.

If you are not this ready, you can wait longer and think about it. Or you can keep reading. There's never an easy time to change habits, but following along with the small behavior changes at the beginning of this book should make you feel more ready and more convinced you WILL starting exercising more.

I begin by talking about why it's so hard for people to maintain an exercise habit nowadays. And I end with how to keep exercising and not give-up particularly after all your hard work with this book. In between, you will work through a series of self-management skills, chapter by chapter. They include what and how to keep a record of exercise, scheduling your exercise to fit into your lifestyle, controlling events that interfere with exercise, creating a helpful attitude, making your environment conducive for physical activity, encouraging people to be supportive, overcoming apprehension and resistance to exercise, and using self-motivation strategies.

Several chapters will help you modify the qualities of your exercise including how often you exercise, for how long, how intense, and what types of exercise you do. You will learn psychological techniques to follow these recommendations. While this might sound like advice on fitness training that I promised not to give, the real purpose behind these chapters is for you to deepen your exercise habit.

Your goal at the beginning should be to just start moving a little more and to not worry about the quality of your exercise. The few chapters on refining the quality of exercise appear later because at the beginning, basic motivation is more important.

This book is a workbook. You will read the psychological concepts and examples of how they apply to exercise. Then you will assess yourself with forms and worksheets to see where you stand with respect to the self-management skills. To help you concretely, you will read examples of how to change and the challenges to making those changes. I include information that could be in a psychology textbook. If you learn those concepts, you'll make a stronger exercise habit.

The disadvantage of a self-help workbook is there is no one to supervise you and hold you accountable. The advantage is you are in control and can work at your own pace. You will get more from this book if you use it correctly. Do not read the book all at once. Use it as a step-by-step guide. The chapters are in a sequence, introducing concepts in sync with expected increases in exercise. Do not switch to the next chapter until you really have put the new self-management skill into action. It's up to you to be honest. Go through the motions of completing the forms and practicing the skill. Then work on the next one. Completing one chapter per week beginning with Chapter 3, would be a good pace because that corresponds with the time needed to strengthen a habit.

Going in order from Chapter 3 to 5 is especially important because they cover the basics on measuring and scheduling exercise. Thereafter, the order is logical, but if you are having trouble with something addressed by a later chapter, it is okay to read ahead so long as you resume the book in order. Of course, you can return to the past chapters repeatedly as you need to review and sharpen your skills. In the long run, the book or individual chapters should be revisited when you encounter trouble. I think of this book as a program that can be spread over months, as much time as it takes for a real habit to develop.

How Health Professionals Can Use This Book

Most health professionals who want their patients or clients to exercise more are not exercise or behavior change experts, nor do they have the time to intervene adequately with exercise problems. A simple solution would be to assign this book. With just a little support and follow-up, the reader should benefit much more than from the brief exercise messages that practitioners can give. I also recommend that health professionals use it themselves as a clinical guidebook on how to talk to their clients or patients about exercise and what advice to give.

Health and wellness practitioners are an important gateway for triggering health behavior change in the whole population. Here are some clinicians who can put this book to work in their practice. 1) Dietitians need to increase exercise to produce weight loss, but most diet books and even behavioral weight control books are weak on exercise. 2) Primary care practitioners (family doctors, internal medicine physicians, geriatricians, pediatricians, and nurse practitioners) know that almost all chronic medical problems are improved with exercise, but they have so little time to give more than a one-minute message to exercise. 3) Physical therapists teach exercise in the clinic, but patients do not necessarily follow-through when unsupervised at home. 4) Personal trainers are strong on how to become fit but weak on getting people to follow-through when personal supervision is over. 5) Fitness centers lose most new members because they do not address the problem of keeping people committed to exercise. 6) Mental health professionals are increasingly aware that exercise is related to psychological health, but they are skilled in therapy for mental health symptoms, not necessarily for lifestyle change.

Regardless of the profession, I recommend that you read and use the book yourself. Research shows clinical practitioners are more likely to recommend exercise if they exercise themselves. Personal success with this system will let you give advice and recommend the book confidently.

Chapter 2:
It's Hard to Make Yourself Exercise

We are capable of long and hard physical work. Our heritage equipped our bodies, but our environment, physical and cultural, now encourages us to be physically inactive. Some obstacles to exercise are not your fault, but they must be controlled in order to make yourself exercise.

We Were Born To Exercise

Today we must consciously schedule exercise into our daily routine whereas before the modern era, it was triggered by necessity. Physical activity was necessary for survival; physical inactivity would lead to death.

Until agriculture began around 10,000 years ago, people spent most of their time hunting, foraging and preparing food. Without a way to store it, looking for food was daily work. Early men and women in hunter-gatherer societies walked many miles every day. In addition to creating physical endurance, daily work made people strong. Over time people underwent physical changes to make them capable of larger and larger amounts of physical work. Our body type and capacity for physical work were established in our genes during this hunter-gatherer era. Our heredity has not changed significantly since.

During the transition to agriculture, some of the physical hardship was reduced by getting food from domesticated plants and animals instead of having to roam greater distances. Still, life involved a great deal of physical activity to cultivate food, fetch water and so on. It was not until the industrial revolution a couple hundred years ago that people (in advanced countries) became sedentary because machines replaced labor-intensive jobs and the new city life required less moving around. But human bodies were not designed to be sedentary.

Biologically the human body depended on lots of physical activity for proper health and now modern humans who lack activity suffer from chronic diseases they would not have had thousands of years ago. Lack of exercise contributes to diabetes, obesity, and cardiovascular disease and beyond these increasingly prevalent health problems, there is almost no illness, psychological problem, or ache or pain that cannot be prevented or helped by exercise. There even is a connection between exercise and better cognitive function during later adulthood. We are capable of the same intensely active lifestyle and healthy physiques of our cavemen ancestors. Physical, genetic capacity is not the problem. We were born to exercise.

Why Don't We Exercise?

We were born to rest. We were designed to exercise, but to survive we also had a drive to be inactive and rest. There was no point in burning up all their calories looking for food when there was none to be found. Early humans had to conserve energy and supplies of calories stored in body fat by not engaging in needless activity, especially during periods of famine. Otherwise they could starve. And when searching for food, it had to be done efficiently – expending the least amount of physical energy over the least amount of time possible with the greatest certainty of getting food. Our nervous system was hard wired to fine tune unconsciously even simple body movements to keep the energy cost as low as possible.

Generally, there was more need than not for our ancestors to be physically active. But not every day was an exercise day. Hunting and foraging cycled with inactivity so the body could recover from hard physical work. Without rest, humans wouldn't be able to go on the next hunt. Modern athletes, who follow an exercise training plan, deliberately schedule rest or recovery days. Our ancestors didn't have to schedule rest days. Their drive to rest was automatic. If left to conscious thinking and reasoning, they wouldn't have survived.

Being lazy is human nature not a moral defect. We inherited the need to be inactive and shouldn't feel guilty. Yes, unfortunately nowadays the environment allows us to be inactive more than ever before. To overcome that unhealthy influence we must overcome the instinct to rest when we don't really need to rest.

The environment doesn't make us exercise. Daily activities of humans used to depend completely on physical exertion by the individual. Now physical activity has been engineered out of our lives to the point that it's hardly a requirement for daily living. Nutrition hardly needs physical activity because agricultural industry and modern food distribution bring food to us. Even food preparation, cooking and cleanup are declining as people eat out more often.

Most people live in urban areas where work and daily life are sedentary compared to how it used to be living on a farm. Almost everyone commutes to work or errands by private car. Just a very small percent walk or ride a bicycle. In a big city or high-density residential neighborhood, people can get to public transportation, neighborhood shopping and entertainment on foot. Whereas in most suburbs, neighborhoods are spread out. Supermarkets and big stores are further away from home and work commutes are much longer, consequently people tend to drive everywhere. Even children are walking or riding bikes to school less. Among people who do commute by walking, the average distance is less than a mile.

Urban design puts automobiles and buses over human powered

transportation. When bike lanes, school-safe riding routes, recreation paths, sidewalks, pedestrian walkways, and public lighting are added, walking and riding bikes increase. Physical activity is triggered by environmental cues almost automatically. A simple example: put a cute sign in a shopping mall suggesting the stairs, not escalator. A lot more people use stairs. Ironically, it's hard nowadays to find stairs in public buildings.

Labor saving devices and computerized technologies have eliminated physical activity at home and work. Power garden equipment, snow blowers, and household appliances cut down on housework. Every little bit of labor saving makes a physical difference. The electric wine bottle opener deprives one of a small calorie burn and wrist strengthening exercise. Power equipment and robotics in manufacturing and the building trades have reduced physical labor. Shopping by Internet where a purchase and doorstep delivery deprives one of having to burn some calories by walking around the parking lot and store or carrying purchases into the car and house. Electronic communication means one doesn't have to walk to the mailbox with a letter or even to the next cubicle at work to speak to your co-worker. Participation in physical recreation has declined as people spend more time entertaining themselves via the Internet, social media and spectator sports.

The radical reduction in physical activity after prehistoric humans did not finish with the machine age. In the past fifty years alone, people have been burning hundreds fewer calories per day working and taking care of the home. And low energy recreation is taking up more of our time when we could be outdoors and active. The environment and technology might be to blame for this, but the solution depends on individual self-control. Needing self-control is not meant to imply non-exercisers have a willpower or problem inside. People blame themselves too much for poor health habits. The decline in physical activity is better explained by outside, environmental factors: less demand for physical activity and fewer role models for exercise. But to increase physical activity, you indeed will have to ignore what the rest of the world does. You will have to let go of some convenient and easy ways and do some things the old fashion way, by hand or foot.

Most people do not exercise. Let's begin with some basic facts about how many people exercise. It turns out the rate is so low that to exercise is abnormal, at least in the statistical sense. We will see how this makes people exercise even less.

How many people exercise? A standard for adequate exercise is set by the Centers for Disease Control and Prevention (CDC) of the US Department of Health and Human Services. The current one is 30 minutes of moderately intense aerobic activity most days of the week. Most days is translated concretely as five days a week for a total of two and one-half hours of aerobic exercise. Moderately intense refers to a slight to moderate increase in breathing or heart rate or light sweating and is maintained for at least ten minutes without stopping. Strengthening exercise, which refers to weight training or calisthenics, should be done on two days per week. An alternative is 75 minutes of vigorous exercise (e.g. running or some aerobic exercise with heavy breathing that makes it difficult to speak), plus strengthening exercise.

Do you exercise this much? And the answer for the whole country is .... Less than 20 percent of adults age 18 years and older exercise adequately. And nearly one-half of adults get absolutely no leisure time physical activity. Not much better, just 25 percent of adolescents meet the CDC's recommendation for children - one-hour daily (translated as five hours per week) of moderate to vigorous activity (large increases in breathing or heart rate). Those statistics are based on answers to questionnaires. But people overestimate desirable behavior. Looking at activity in people who are measured objectively with a physical device like a fitness tracker, the actual rate of exercise is even lower, maybe as low as five percent.

Some non-government health experts say people need even more exercise to be healthy in order to avoid, for example, becoming overweight or obese or in order to lose a substantial amount of weight. A better standard would be an hour a day for a minimum of five hours of exercise per week including some vigorous exercise. They also say, if you would like to slow the aging process and be more youthful later in life, you probably need a much higher dose of vigorous exercise – more than twice the CDC recommendation. Indeed, some countries other than the United States target five hours of exercise in their public health recommendations. Given that most people do not even meet the CDC "lighter" exercise recommendation, a five-hour minimum of moderate or two and one-half hours of vigorous exercise would categorize almost all adult Americans as inadequate exercisers.

Politics and common sense sometimes rule health standards more than science in order to translate them into public action. The CDC cut point for exercise time is the amount needed to lower risk for diabetes and heart disease. You can argue that there is a lot more to health than having less chance of these two diseases. In older adults it includes not losing cognitive functioning or becoming physically disabled. Or you can argue that a lower exercise standard, even less than the CDC standard, is a good start on health and is less intimidating and more doable because people are so inactive right now. But the psychology of goal setting would predict that any standard no matter how low could discourage instead of encourage exercise. That's because too many people react to goals with an all-or-nothing attitude: "If I don't exercise that much, I might as well not even bother to exercise at all." Regardless of which numbers you choose, if the purpose of an exercise standard is to encourage people to be more physically active, the sad reality is hardly anyone knows the specifics of these recommendations anyway.

Exercise in different populations. Briefly, in regard to race and gender, African Americans, and American Latinos and Asians exercise less and are more likely to not exercise at all compared to white non-Hispanics. Cultural, educational and economic issues underlie this difference. Girls and women exercise less than boys and men and start giving-up exercise earlier. Culturally transmitted sex role behavior explains this difference.

People with some health problems are less likely to exercise: smokers, overweight and obese persons, the physically disabled, and people with psychological or medical problems. People with health problems need exercise the most. But ill health and other unhealthy behavior make it more difficult to exercise. It's a vicious cycle of physical inactivity and worsening health.

Across adulthood, people tend to behave healthier as they grow older. This is evident by trends in smoking, alcohol use, healthy eating, safe sex, wearing seat belts, having a primary care provider, health screening (e.g. blood pressure and cholesterol checks, and colonoscopy), and medication (e.g. taking high blood pressure medication as prescribed). All are better as people age. The only health behavior or risk factor that becomes worse is exercise! The prevalence of exercise declines steadily from 30 percent of young adults to eleven percent of adults 65 years and over.

Older people who never smoked wouldn't wake up one day and say, "I think I'll start smoking cigarettes." Yet by middle age people start giving up exercise.

Exercise habits become more similar in married couples as they age. If one spouse quits exercise, the other one probably will too. It's a pity, because older people can reduce their risk for disease and slow the aging process by exercising even after years of not having exercised.

Ethnic minorities, women, overweight persons, the disabled and chronically ill, and older persons, in addition to exercising less, also spend more time being sedentary or completely inactive (sitting) which we will see predicts poor health apart from the effect of exercise.

People don't exercise because no one else is. Looking at the statistics another way, we know that eighty percent of people do not exercise. That leaves a small minority to serve as role models for healthy behavior. If you are a woman, older adult or member of a racial minority, you might have hardly any peers around you that exercise. On the contrary, almost everyone is modeling how to be sedentary and avoid physical activity. That's the norm. To exercise is abnormal (in the statistical sense). Of course, certain occupation and education levels and regions of the country include lots more who exercise. People usually want to conform to what is regarded as normal and accepted behavior in their own immediate social environment even if it's not good for you. When there's little social encouragement, going against the norm takes determination and even courage.

Most non-exercisers admit that exercise is good for your health and they want to exercise. That doesn't mean people around you will celebrate if you abandon the sedentary way of life. They might disapprove or interfere, instead. Negative messages about exercising are expressed in disdainful stereotypes of exercisers, jokes, and put-downs. To the outside world, dedicated exercisers can be perceived as compulsive, vain, self-centered, anorexic or extreme. To criticize what you secretly wish that you could do is a thinly disguised defense mechanism to feel okay about your choice.

Starting to exercise might be a social challenge too. But I hope you will have lots of people to cheer you on. Tips on encouraging support follow in a later chapter.

Exercise is hard. Exercise is good for you but it feels bad before it feels or does any good. How do you feel when exercising? Do you feel tired or sore? Feel stressed? Does sweating bother you? Do you hear yourself breathing loudly? Feel out of shape? Feel awkward? Sensations from exercising can feel really unpleasant even frightening and are not a reward for your hard effort.

You might say exercise is going to be your new priority, but what happens when you face the reality of exercise taking time away from more pleasant or more pressing activities? Does it seem that you don't have time to exercise? Do you feel like you are gaining or losing something?

To make matters more discouraging, do you notice big changes in your fitness or physique after a week of good exercise? No, the improvements are longer term, not immediate.

Altogether, it's reasonable for people to feel like exercise is a loss, or speaking technically, a punishment rather than a reward. The more unfit or overweight you are, the more like a punishment it can feel. No wonder it's so hard to get going. Proper self-management techniques will help you survive the initial difficult weeks and keep going until exercise is something you look forward to.

Habit change is hard. Are you so enthusiastic that you feel burned-out from exercising too much at the beginning? Do you increase exercise so slowly that you aren't improving? Do you give excuses too often for not exercising? Are you having trouble letting go of other pastimes in order to keep exercise on your schedule? Do you give-in too much to time demands? Are you too lax in keeping track of your progress? Are other people talking you out of exercise? Do you feel like too much of a klutz to be physical? Do you have some kind of self-image problem during workouts? Do you tell yourself it's hopeless when you have a setback? Is your exercise program a set-up for failure? Do you feel like a failure? Do you think you just don't have will power?

There are so many problems to overcome. Inability to stay motivated is the hardest part of changing health habits. Unfortunately, most people don't give themselves enough time to work through all their exercise barriers. On average, people quit in two months after trying to lose weight or exercise. If you signed-up for a fitness center and go for less than a couple months, have exercise and going to the gym become habits? No. Habits are behaviors that are deeply engrained and strengthened by repetition over a long period of time. Habit is the point you reach when behavior seems to occur automatically without having to consciously decide or talk yourself into doing it. That's hardly the case at the beginning. After a couple weeks in the fitness center, you might say your commitment to exercise has strengthened. You are more determined to keep exercising. You are more optimistic that you won't give-up this time. These are good attitudes, but you haven't exercised often or long enough to make it a habit.

Unfortunately, people interpret quitting exercise as evidence they can't do it. But if you quit early, you haven't given up much. You've only given up the idea or intention to become an exerciser. You quit when exercise was still a weak behavior, when you were at risk for quitting, when the aversive consequences of exercise were greater than the pleasurable consequences. If people were able to not quit for a few months in a row, the quit rate would be much lower. That's because by that time, the whole exercise ritual would be learned, non-exercise behavior would be unlearned, and exercise would feel physically and mentally easier. To not exercise would start feeling unnatural.

Too bad people wait so long to make another attempt – five years on average. That compounds the problem by slowing down the learning process. Most health behaviors are changed over time with repeated attempts. At some point for successful people, something clicks and the behavior is established. So ideally you won't delay and you will start another exercise attempt now and try to deal with the problems that interfered the last time.

Most causes of suffering or quitting exercise can be controlled by cognitive and behavioral self-management techniques. People can learn these techniques and learn how to survive the first months to the point when it's a habit. There is no better time than now.

Dieting is more popular than exercise. Most people are not exercising. But at any one time, most people are dieting. I'm talking about dieting because most resolutions to exercise begin with wanting to lose weight. It turns out that weight control programs and books contain much more information and instruction on changing eating behavior, especially reducing calories, than on increasing exercise. Popular media is filled with commentaries on changing the diet. Internet searches on diet and obesity vastly outnumber searches on inactivity and obesity. The same lopsided bias exists in the scientific literature. Ironically, over the past couple decades Americans have been eating fewer calories but have become more overweight because they've reduced physical activity. But if you increase exercise and remain overweight, your chance of serious disease still decreases significantly.

So, why has exercise taken a back seat to dieting for physical fitness?

It's easier. The simplest answer is that it takes a lot less time and energy to eat less food than it does to go outside and be physical. It's the easier way to tip the balance between calories eaten and calories burned. For you to save 300 calories by substituting nonfat frozen yogurt for regular ice cream takes much less effort than to reduce the same amount of calories by walking three miles. People want a quick fix and to not suffer. Why not eat less instead of being uncomfortable and inconvenienced by exercise. It's the easier way out for weight loss.

In the beginning when the dieter can make simple calorie cuts like eating yogurt instead of ice cream every day for a week, one could lose almost a pound. You'd have to walk 21 miles in a week for the same weight loss. But for a variety of reasons calorie reduction by itself becomes less effective over time. Long-term weight loss is better with exercise added and physical health in general is better. Above all, for the sake of habit change, dieting takes something away – it's a deprivation approach, whereas exercise adds something positive (after the initial phase).

There's more psychological attention on food. Psychologists and experts also have mistakenly promoted food reduction as the best or only solution. Going way back to the psychoanalyst Sigmund Freud is his notion that overeating is symptomatic of a deeper psychological problem that comes out in the form of excessive oral behavior. It can lead to obesity, which some psychologists explained as a pathological need for nurturance. But since overeating is obviously unhealthy, the overeater also must have a self-destructive streak. Over time food weirdly has become regarded as both self-love and self-hate. With psychological overtones of an addiction and a struggle between pleasure and denial, the alcoholic's

12-step program adopted the food issue and "Overeaters Anonymous" was born in which participants can testify they have no control over food.

We're obsessed with food and fascinated by behavior like compulsive binge eating, although objectively, declining activity and physical labor are also responsible for weight and other health problems. Is exercise simply not as interesting psychologically as why we put so much food in our mouths? When was the last time you heard a good theory about why some people hate to sweat? Isn't sedentary behavior self-destructive too? Shouldn't people be a little more anxious about their relationship with exercise? Don't people also need help with their relationships with their physical selves, to deal with the struggle between sloth and fitness? How many in Overeaters Anonymous have no motivation to exercise? Where are the Underexercisers Anonymous meetings? I'm half kidding, but the psychology of exercise truly needs more attention.

Health professionals are not necessarily good role models. Health professionals who work in weight control programs and in primary care medicine are among those in the best position to advise people to exercise. In fact, a straightforward message along with a couple tips can motivate patients to start exercising. Yet many patients who are sedentary are not encouraged to exercise by their doctors. Patients who are really overweight or physically impaired need the most encouragement, but receive even less because physicians typically are more pessimistic or unskilled to deal with them. Psychologists and dieticians typically recommend a couple hours of exercise per week to their overweight patients, even though much more is needed to produce a substantial weight loss. Why don't they encourage four, five, six or more hours per week? Why don't they encourage exercise everyday? The answer is simply that health professionals struggle with the same personal obstacles to exercise that we all do. Most of my colleagues who directed weight control programs at other universities of course encouraged exercise, but they were not passionate exercisers themselves. Indeed, the average primary care provider does not exercise enough either. If you haven't made exercise a major part of your life, how can you expect your patients to?

Conclusion

This chapter has been about how our environment, physical and cultural, determines physical activity. I think it's encouraging to remember that biologically, genetically people are capable of lots and lots of physical activity even though our environment does not require it. There is an analogy in the field of health about the cause of disease that applies to capacity to exercise: "Genetics loads the gun, but the environment pulls the trigger." A translation is: genetics prepares our body to exercise, but the environment must encourage it. Self-management is the process of changing our environment and our reactions to it, exactly what is needed to realize our potential for fitness.

Chapter 3:
Get Started With Self-Monitoring

Your assignment for Week 1 is to keep an exercise record every day. You will record the type of exercise you did and the amount of time you spent exercising. The purpose is to learn how to self-monitor and to take a baseline on your physical activity in a typical week. Don't skip ahead to the next assignment - yes, I know you want to start your new habit today. Sorry. If you're serious about changing behavior, the first step is to measure the behavior, rather than to try increasing it immediately. Although you shouldn't consciously exercise more than normal, you might find that self-monitoring automatically makes you exercise more anyway, because in addition to being an assessment tool, self-monitoring is a motivation tool. Self-monitoring is an on-going requirement after the first week. This chapter will help you effectively record and use statistics on your exercise.

What Activity To Record

Now what counts as exercise? Any physical activity performed intentionally for physical fitness or recreation goes on your record. Exercise walks, cycling, weight training, yoga, and are clear examples of leisure time physical activity that should be recorded. Exercise does not need to be aerobic or intense to the point of sweating or a big increase in heart rate or breathing to go on the record. Leisurely exercise counts too. Muscle strengthening exercise counts.

There are some types of physical activity that do not go on the record. Walking while shopping I'm afraid, doesn't count. Well, it counts for your body, but not for the record. Walking on the job, washing the car, and mowing the lawn are great for the body too. But all these are activities of daily living, already part of your lifestyle. What you do now in daily life is not enough to be fit, control your weight, or have fun being physical. Otherwise you wouldn't be reading this book.

The purpose of this book is to help you increase your physical activity beyond what you already do. Daily chores normally cannot be avoided and already are done by habit. Whereas fitness exercise for most people is regarded as optional. It's harder to make yourself exercise for the sake of exercise. That is the behavior you are trying to increase, not chores, which already are strongly motivated by needing to function normally. As you will understand later, another purpose of recording your behavior is to increase it. Therefore, your exercise record must focus on real exercise, so that it will stimulate increases in the correct target behavior.

Sometimes it is hard to decide if something is exercise or an activity of daily living because the difference can be more mental than physical; it can depend on your reason for the activity. Here are some examples. Walking while shopping may not be exercise (on your record), but walking to the supermarket instead of driving for the sake of the workout counts as exercise. Mall walking and window-shopping for the sake of an exercise walk counts on your record. If circumstances are such that you have to walk to all your errands, say you live in the inner city and rarely drive, do not record your normal daily commuting time on foot. That walking already is built into your daily function. On the other hand, if you typically drive everywhere and start walking to work or to the store in order to get your workout, even though it's more time consuming and inconvenient, record those walks on your exercise record.

Here is another example of an exception I once made. A patient of mine did practically nothing but knit and read until one day she decided to the shock of her family she would take over mowing the lawn. She was adamant that if she were going to be more physical it would be for a useful purpose. Indeed, mowing the lawn was for her a triumph of motivation over being sedentary– and it went on her exercise record.

Some older adults gradually restrict their daily activity so much, they hardly ever get out of the house. Getting out of the house to do anything, even by car leads to more walking, lifting, moving. If you break out of a disability lifestyle and deliberately make yourself shop or visit, it's okay to keep track of that walking time, because you're accomplishing a health behavior change. Later you can worry about adding a more formal exercise.

Of all the complaints I got, most were for not giving credit for activities of daily living. People want to think they're getting more exercise than they really are. They want to look good on paper. But be honest and record real exercise, the kind of activity you know is for the sake of physical recreation and fitness. That is the target behavior. It should not be difficult to recognize when you deliberately make some practical chore to double as exercise beyond what you normally would do. Otherwise, doing more chores is a side effect of more exercise and is a bonus even if it doesn't go on your record.

How To Record Your Exercise

Record the time spent exercising in minutes or hours and minutes. Use a clock or watch or activity timer and check the time when you start your walk – not when you start to put your shoes on, and at the end – when you arrive at the front door – not when you have arrived undressed at the shower. Within reason, only include actual exercise time – time you're moving. If your 23-minute walk included a one-minute chat with the neighbor, it's okay to write 23 minutes. But if you go skiing and spend a couple hours in the cafeteria, deduct that time from the total time of your outing. Record accurately; don't guess or round off. If all your walks are 20, 30, 40 minutes, you are estimating, not measuring.

You want to know the exact time spent exercising in a week, because to strengthen that behavior, you may need to make small, gradual increases in time, maybe by just a few minutes. Estimations will make it difficult for you to schedule systematic increases in exercise.

Self-monitoring is an exercise in honesty. You can't change a behavior without looking at yourself honestly. Self-deception interferes with self-change, because you can't change something that doesn't exist. It is better to trust the watch than your subjective sense of time because, not surprisingly, people concerned about a behavior typically are not accurate in estimating it. In which way are people inaccurate? You guessed it; in the direction that makes them feel good – people are more likely to overestimate than underestimate the time they exercise.

Exercise is a desirable behavior. Overeating is an undesirable behavior and people concerned about their weight typically underestimate their calorie consumption. There is an unconscious bias toward estimating exercise behavior in the direction of your ideal or expectation. Be an honest and accurate recorder. This improves control over the behavior and promotes self-acceptance.

Daily record. Here is an example of a daily exercise record to use at this time (Figure 3.1), followed by a blank form that you can reproduce (Figure 3.2). Or make your own form, use a journal, or track your exercise with a computer program or an app on your smart phone or tablet. At the end of the week, add the number of days on which you exercised and the number of minutes or hours and minutes. As you advance in how to make an exercise habit, there will be other things to record in your diary, but at this stage, do not create an exercise sheet that reads like a novel. There may be many interesting things going on in your life that affect whether you go out the door to be physical, but for now, just the numbers please. These numbers on time and frequency are the only concrete behavioral facets of exercise that you need to change for now. Stay focused on these numbers. The quality of your exercise is not important at this time.

Digital activity trackers that measure speed and steps or mileage, for example, could be useful when we start talking about varying exercise intensity. Like any form of self-monitoring, they can motivate you to take more steps or more miles. That is a good thing. But the total time you spend exercising influences the strength of your exercise habit, as you will understand better later. That's why you need that information. Steps taken by walking are not perfectly associated with time. But time is a unit of measurement that can be applied to different types of exercise, so you can combine the "dose" of exercise you get from steps or miles with some other activity that might be measured differently like vertical feet skiing. So, I ask you to please calculate these measures of time in addition to or in place of any automated activity monitoring you might already use.

week starting Jan 1	exercise	time
Monday	walk the dog	16 min
Tuesday	stretch & yoga walk to market	24 min 12 min
Wednesday	0	0

Figure 3.1 A daily record of exercise includes the type of activity and the exact amount of time.

week starting	exercise (if more than one bout of exercise, list separately)	time
Monday		
Tuesday		
Wednesday		
Thursday		
Friday		
Saturday		
Sunday		

number of days with exercise _____   total time _____

Figure 3.2 Honest and accurate recording of exercise is important in order to change your behavior.

Weekly record. The next step is to start a graph of weekly exercise, graphing number of days with exercise and total time spent exercising. The purpose is to have a useful visual representation of your trend over time. Seeing the exercise data summarized week by week is important feedback on your behavior change. There are many characteristics of exercise one could record. For the moment, frequency of exercise – in the form of days per week, and total time are the two most important. These are the features of exercise that you will be modifying in the next month or so.

Check the example graph below (Figure 3.3). Notice there are two lines of data, one for hours and one for days per week. Put a data point for each at the end of the first week and later, connect the weekly data points to separate hours from days and to see the trend over time. Estimate the location of the data point as accurately as possible. The horizontal lines on this chart are in half-hour increments. So, three and one-quarter hours of exercise would have to be marked in-between two of the lines as shown for week four on the graph.

I labeled the first column of data to the far left as Week 0, your first week of recording, because this is your "baseline" week, before you should start changing your exercise time. If your total exercise time and days are zero, fine. Record that zero. The good news is you have a lot of room to improve.

The example in Figure 3.3 is the average of hundreds of people, which makes the trend over time look fairly smooth and steady. Any one person's graph might look much more erratic, fluctuating between a week with hardly any exercise and some with hours and hours. I am not showing you this graph as a model to follow, week by week. Yours might have lots of ups and downs.

Reproduce the blank graph further below (Figure 3.4) for your own use or make your own with graph paper or a spreadsheet program or use an app that summarizes exercise in a graph or table. Write the dates for the beginning of each week along the bottom. Dates on the graph will help you see the relation between time of year and the amount you exercise. This could be useful information to understand circumstances that affect your exercise.

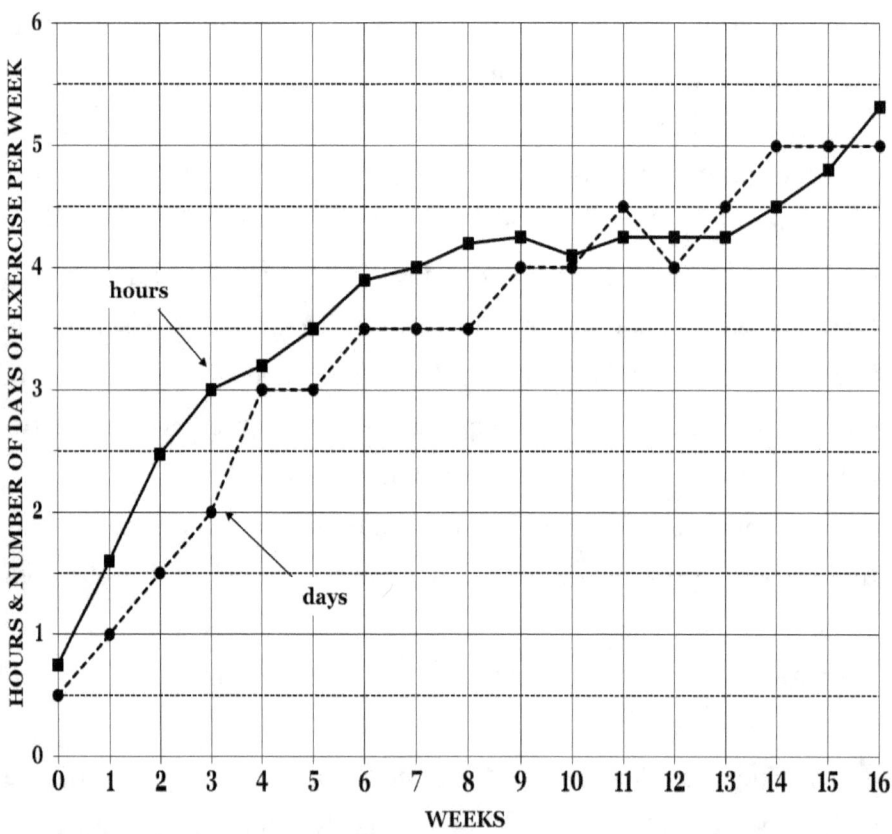

Figure 3.3 A graph of the number of days on which you exercised and the total time you spent exercising gives you helpful visual feedback on your progress. People who follow this program are able to make the steady increases shown on this graph.

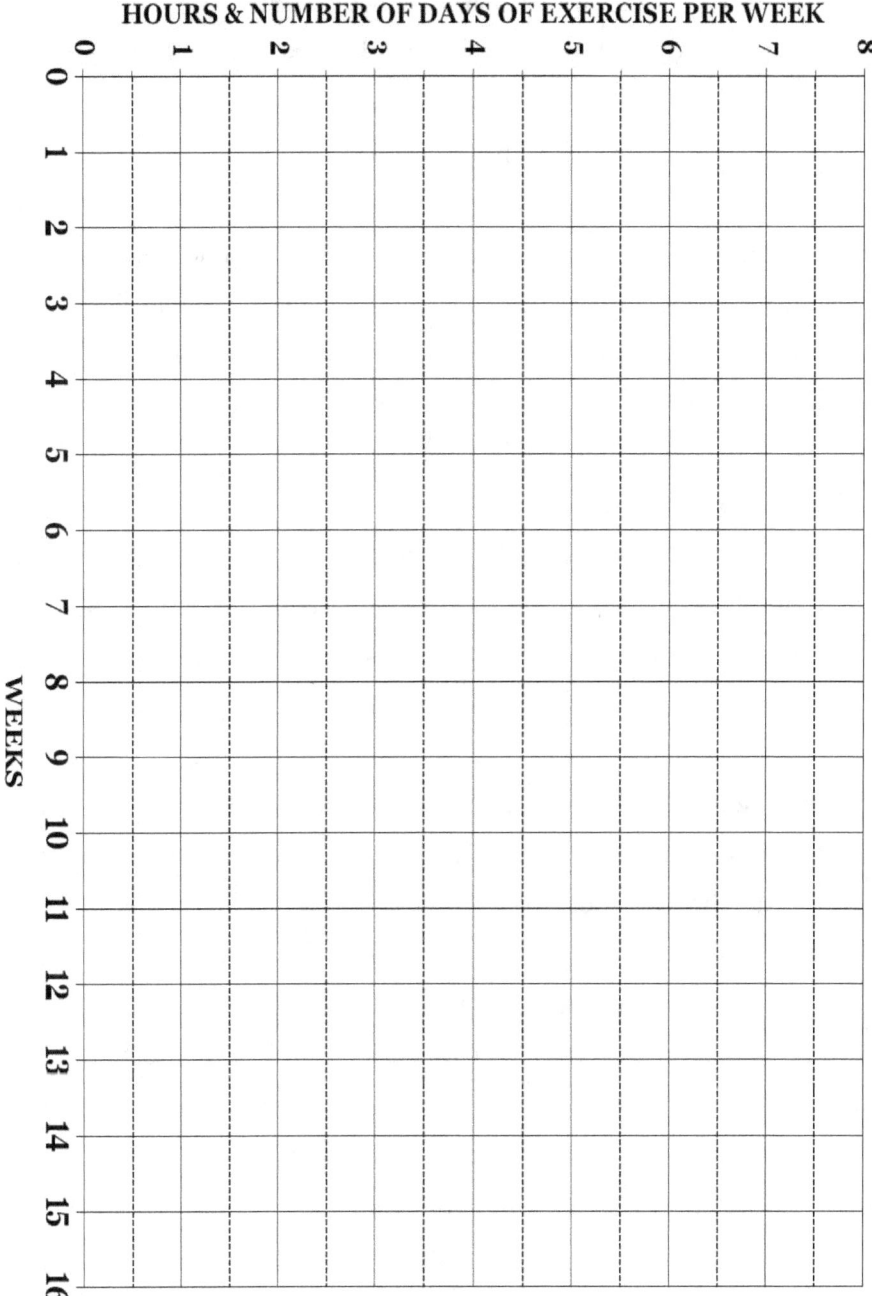

Figure 3.4 Use a graph like this to start recording number of days and time per week, using a separate line for each.

How Much Do People Increase Their Exercise?

Look back at the example exercise graph in Figure 3.3. It is based on the actual results of over 500 people in my former University of Vermont Weight Control Program. Each data point is the average or median (middle score of all the people) week by week during the four-month program. The participants on average, weighed 248 pounds, were in their mid-forties and typically had some physical limitations and medical problems such as diabetes and other cardiac risk factors associated with their overweight. Most were sedentary at the beginning and not only were they physically inactive, but most of them felt intimidated by exercise.

There are some important lessons in this exercise graph which we should touch on now. The good news is that even people with a lot of challenges can substantially increase their exercise using the behavioral principles in this book. The bad news is, it takes time: in this example four months to reach a reasonably active lifestyle. In addition, the average result of 5.32 hours per week in 5 days of exercise, although great for people who overcame a lot of adversity, is still below the goal I will set forth in this book of 6 hours in 6 days. It can take even longer than a few months for many people to reach that goal.

Notice that people typically increase exercise quickly in the first month. I think they are enthusiastic at the beginning and discover that to exercise a couple hours per week is manageable. Afterward, for the next couple months, exercise increases slowly and even levels out for a while. Although it seems like people stop progressing, actually this is progress toward a new habit because habit is formed through repeated practice. I suspect that when people reach a moderate amount of exercise, without consciously knowing it, they need time to stick with that level until it feels easier and more routine – like a habit.

Toward the end of these four months, they are ready to make another increase in exercise. I think it takes until then to adjust physically and psychologically to a larger amount of physical activity and to solve the various practical challenges of changing ones lifestyle. If we drew a graph further out in time, a year or longer, we probably would see that dedicated exercisers on their way up in fitness, go through cycles of increasing, holding steady, and increasing again until they reach some optimal level.

Suggestions for your exercise increase over time. Let's translate this trend for increasing exercise into suggestions for you. Take advantage of your enthusiasm and try to increase steadily during the first couple months of this program. Even small increases in minutes add up. Then don't be surprised if you experience a lull and you stay around the same level for a while. You may need to do this in order to adjust to the change you've made. Pushing yourself too quickly might be stressful and cause you to quit. Then work on reaching an even greater amount of exercise time. In chapters to come you will find tips on how to keep making progress. You're just beginning. Do not worry way in advance about how much you will have to exercise in months from now.

The Psychology Of Self-Monitoring

The definition of self-monitoring is the act of observing and recording one's own behavior. These are two different skills. A person can be good at recognizing his or her behavior, but finds a diary to be a nuisance or does not want to see his or her performance in writing. Another person might have no problem recording in a diary, but is poor at self-observation, because he or she estimates too much instead of accurately measuring excrcise. Both skills, observing and recording, are important for creating your exercise habit.

Having asked you to start by recording your typical week, don't be surprised if recording exercise makes you exercise more. That's because behavior is reactive to self-monitoring. If you pay more attention to a behavior, you consciously or unconsciously will modify it. Happily, any changes in behavior that are triggered by self-monitoring tend to be in the desired direction. People in weight control programs, for example, tend to consume fewer calories when they count them and exercise more when they record it. Why? Self-monitoring forces you to compare your actual behavior with your desired or ideal behavior. People are motivated to live up to their ideal, especially when given feedback about their performance. If you can't help but be a little more active in the first week because you're measuring yourself, okay, but don't consciously increase beyond normal.

Self-monitoring is the number one technique that people naturally use to maintain or refocus their control over health habits. In long-term weight control especially, people who successfully maintain weight loss for years say they keep a food diary, if not continuously, at least when their habits start slipping. And among graduates of my weight control program, the most frequent technique people used to re-focus or correct their fitness was to start recording again.

Use your exercise record, not just for information, but also for change. Self-monitoring not only is a tool to analyze and understand your behavior, but it is a powerful technique to change your behavior, usually in the direction you desire.

How To Improve Your Self-Monitoring

Self-monitoring is simple but not easy for everyone. Here are some suggestions to make your self-monitoring more reliable and effective.

1. Record immediately after the behavior in order to be more

accurate. People tend to underestimate undesirable behavior and overestimate desirable behavior even more when they delay recording. Filling in your diary at the end of the week is not okay.

2. You can even record before you begin in order to make a commitment to exercise. For instance, you check your diary and see that today you need to do a longer walk to balance it with the shorter walks you already had this week. So you write "Walk – 60 minutes" in your record before you leave for your workout. A plan in writing makes it more likely you'll follow through, because a written, concrete intention is more powerful than simply thinking about it. Recording a behavior beforehand facilitates behavior change.

3. Use cues to remind you to record. The sight of your record is the best cue, so keep your exercise record with you and visible. A reminder cue can be anything else in your environment or daily routine that you consistently associate with recording. For instance, you might update your diary every morning when you sit to do your computer chores. Or you might keep your exercise record in your appointment book or phone where you already are recording something else like your schedule. The key is to use the same cue consistently. Associate recording with some time or place so that recording exercise will be triggered automatically.

4. Use your record to remind you to exercise. The sight of your diary is a cue to record, but also a cue to exercise. Use it to your advantage. When you see the diary, consciously say something to yourself that strengthens your intention to exercise that day, for instance, "Oh yeah, I need to plan when I'll go for my walk today." You should have as many exercise cues in your environment as possible. The diary is the handiest. Make it a strong reminder to get your workout. (See the Chapter on "Cue Your Exercise" for more ideas.)

5. Record everyday, even if your exercise time is zero. The reason...people are more likely to change if they record every day or every instance of the behavior, not just when they have good days or good behavior. In weight control, sometimes people skip their food diary when they've overeaten or don't weigh themselves when they think they've gained weight. Avoidance of recording to save face is self-defeating. Make yourself record on non-exercise days and write that zero in the diary. (See Figure 3.1 for an example.) Non-exercise IS a behavior, a behavior you are trying to decrease. Seeing a zero on the record is feedback that hopefully will create some discomfort on your part and inspire you to not have a zero the next day. To not write a zero is not facing reality.

6. Be happy about recording even if you're not happy about your exercise. If you start giving excuses for not recording or think too negatively about the results on your record, work on your self-talk. You could think of some positive aspect of recording instead of dwelling on the negative. For instance, tell yourself: "I'm doing a good job of keeping a diary", "The best way to change is to write down everything I do", "Recording my exercise time will help me increase it", "It's a good thing to look at myself honestly". If you're struggling, deliberately repeat some helpful self-talk every time you record until your attitude has changed. Inaccurate recording is often due to wanting to avoid facing reality. See the chapter on Clean-up Your Self-Talk for instruction on modifying negative thoughts.

7. Use your record as a cue to reward exercise. Writing in the record is an opportunity to tell yourself something positive about your exercise, such as, "Great, I got my workout today." Simply seeing your exercise in writing can be a nice self-reward for your work. If you fell short of your exercise plan, recording still should be accompanied by

some helpful self-statement such as, "I missed today, but I have a definite plan for tomorrow.

8. People are more likely to self-monitor if they make a verbal commitment to other people. If you want to motivate yourself to record, tell someone that you are keeping an exercise diary. Likewise, self-monitoring is more accurate and consistent when people know their work will be checked. Consider swapping your exercise record with a friend or turn-in your diary to some supportive person who will encourage you to continue. Some fitness apps on smartphones allow you to friend other people and give them access or notifications of your exercise and nutrition diary. They can post comments to your app.

9. Having a goal for behavior change makes people keep better track of their behavior. That's because a goal is usually more demanding than normal and people want to know when they reach it and can relax. A bonus is that seeing progress toward it in a diary will encourage you to accomplish that goal. So here is another example of a two-way effect in self-monitoring. A goal encourages self-monitoring. Self-monitoring encourages achieving the goal. In Chapter 5 you will learn about setting a goal to increase exercise time.

10. Use a mobile phone app, GPS or fitness tracker that tracks exercise such as a walking, running, or cycling. These programs rely on GPS or body motion to compute the time and distance you move and are even more accurate than looking at a clock or starting and stopping a timer and dramatically more accurate than your own estimate. There are fitness apps that can be used to accurately time all kinds of workouts. For instance, there are yoga apps that present a timed session with a sequence of poses.

If you like gadgets and computer apps, a walking, running, or cycling app that has a lot of pleasing and useful visual information not only gives you data for your diary, but acts like a reward for exercising. Most apps that track movements also calculate the calories you burned. That is another positive feedback for your effort to encourage more exercise.

Daily feedback from an app is not enough. You or your app still needs to put that information into a form that shows changes over time, months of changes in the two main targets of this program – number of days and hours of exercise per week. The graph, like the example of Figure 3.3 should prove you are progressing or make you self-correct if you are not.

The longer you wear or use your activity tracker, the more likely it will become an automatic part of your self-monitoring system. But if you stop using it, as do most people, you probably will need to use a simpler method to measure and record your activity. Going without recording altogether is not an option.

11. Let your diary teach you how much to exercise. Not the first week, but over time the diary and exercise graph should help you associate the amounts and types of exercise that predict your fitness and your feelings about exercise. In weight control, perhaps the most important lesson from an eating diary is how many calories you can eat and still lose weight. Without counting calories or keeping track of food in some way, there is no accurate way to know. In an exercise program, certain amounts of exercise will make you feel fit and strong, whereas lesser amounts will make you feel weak. Certain amounts will give you momentum to exercise a lot more whereas lesser amounts will make you feel lazy. You need an exercise diary, week after week to see these trends.

The Best Way To Change A Behavior, Is To Measure The Behavior

Self-monitoring is a powerful tool for self-knowledge and change. You can use a simple diary as the focal point of your new exercise habit. Increasing the accuracy and completeness of your recording is as important as increasing exercise itself. Be patient. One behavior change will trigger another. Let your diary inspire attentiveness and interest in your physical activity and enjoy the automatic positive effects.

Chapter 4:
Increase Your Exercise Frequency

Your next assignment is to increase your exercise frequency or the number of days in a week that you exercise. The purpose of exercising more often is to speed up your learning and to make exercise a habit. At this stage, how much time you spend exercising, the type of exercise you do, and the quality of that exercise are much less important than the frequency. The best first step to creating a habit is to practice the behavior over and over until it is learned and automatic. In this chapter I will explain how a habit develops and present a schedule for increasing exercise frequency.

Standards For Exercise Frequency

When I started my practice in weight control in the 1970's it was assumed that clogging of the arteries, high cholesterol and high blood pressure were normal, inevitable consequences of aging. But long-term studies eventually showed that certain health habits including exercise predicted which men and women had a greater risk of developing these problems or dying from heart disease. An exercise recommendation of just 20 minutes of aerobic activity three days per week was promoted as enough to reduce the risk.

More than thirty years later, the latest public health recommendation increased the number of recommended days to most or five days per week for about 30 minutes of moderately intense exercise each time. An alternative for people who prefer vigorous exercise is 75 minutes per week, which is most likely to be spread out over a couple days. Because 80 percent of the population falls below these levels, we have to assume that the weekly frequency for most people is very low, perhaps one or two days per week at most.

If you start at zero days per week, getting to a couple days is a good accomplishment and good for your body. But in the long run a low frequency is inefficient for learning and bad for creating a habit. Simply said, if you are exercising two days per week, you are practicing not-exercising five days per week. Which is the stronger habit, to exercise or to not-exercise?

I recommend that you start by trying to reach four days per week of exercise in order to tip the balance toward exercising more often than not. Then I recommend that you reach six days per week. I could push for daily exercise, but I will allow you one day off because realistically in any given week, even the most dedicated people encounter some interference with exercise.

Hopefully I will persuade you that daily or near daily exercise is beneficial and within your grasp if you gradually increase from your starting level.

The Nature Of Habit

Definition of habit. A habit is a recurrent, unconscious pattern of behavior that is acquired through frequent repetition. Let's break apart this definition. Exercise is recurrent – that means you exercise all the time, it's routine like a part of every day, it's a regular, frequent behavior. Exercise is unconscious – you do it automatically without having to analyze whether you should or should not. Because cues in the environment trigger exercise, not much deliberate thinking is required. You just do it. Exercise is a pattern of behavior – it's not just the physical movement involved, but also a sequence of actions leading up to and after the physical effort, the complete exercise ritual and circumstances surrounding it.

Before it's a habit. You might feel stressed or mentally exhausted when you try to make yourself exercise. That's because at the beginning, before exercise is automatic, you use a lot of conscious, mental effort everyday to follow through with your intention. What is the mental process before habit? It starts with you telling yourself that you are going to exercise today. Your mind is made up. This is called intention. Intention is an overall feeling or idea that you will change or perform a certain desired behavior. Then other types of thinking come. One is planning or thinking about the what, when, where, how etc. of your intended exercise. You might also think about how to cope with obstacles that could distract or prevent you from following through. To make progress with behavior change you will have to be vigilant about sticking to your plan and revise it accordingly. The next exercise day you go through all this thinking again. Fortunately, this is a temporary phase and you can expect relief as the habit of exercise becomes stronger.

How a habit is learned. To acquire a habit depends a lot on your approach. People who have a totally random exercise schedule, such as taking a walk here or there when time allows, will have trouble making exercise a strong habit. Most new successful exercisers at the beginning tend to do the same thing over and over; the same walk around the neighborhood, the same set of exercises at the gym, the same exercise class. The new exercise is practiced over and over without much variation in time or place or circumstance. Exercise occurs in a predictable context, like walking the neighborhood with work friends during lunch every day. That context or set of cues in the environment (lunchtime, presence of walking partners, being at work, etc.) becomes a trigger, a reminder to exercise. The more the exerciser practices the association between the environmental cues and exercise, the less thinking will be involved. The exerciser will respond more automatically to the environment. The beauty of habit is to exercise does not take much mental energy.

Advantages Of Frequent Exercise

Frequent practice strengthens habit. How often is often enough to make a strong habit? Theoretically, the more often the stronger is the behavior. Exercise is one behavior that can be practiced very, very often. Let's consider a different behavior that we practice very often - tooth brushing. Tooth brushing is a strong habit for most of us, a routine that we practice daily, maybe even three times a day. Can you remember brushing your teeth this morning? Probably not. You might know you did because you did your usual morning ritual at the bathroom sink, but you probably cannot recall images or sensations of brushing. It's automatic; you just do it without thinking. You don't need to decide if you will brush. Tooth brushing doesn't require a lot of concentration. It's is a powerful habit. If you don't brush, you feel strange.

Let's say one day you read, experts recommend brushing only every other day. What would happen to your habit? You would have to think every morning, is this a tooth brushing day? Did I brush yesterday? Do I feel like brushing today? It's not automatic without conscious thought any longer. Since you don't have to brush every day, since any one day is optional rather than mandatory, it's easier to slip. You might think, "Oh, I'm running late for work. I'll brush tomorrow instead." More and more circumstances that compete with tooth brushing could win because you wouldn't have the expectation that you must. You would have tomorrow as the way out. Tooth brushing would become a weak habit.

Similarly, in the case of exercise, if it's not a daily event, you'll have to decide, is today an exercise day? If you're still struggling with exercise, this gives you the opportunity to think of excuses to not. Chances are if you're busy, the weather is bad, or you're not in the mood, you'll skip that day. You'll have a habit of exercising on the easy days, but not the hard days. Unfortunately, there always are hard days, sometimes a week or two, three weeks of hard days. Then what happens? The frequency of exercise decreases and the habit disappears, because you've trained yourself through prior episodes to not exercise under adversity. You've trained yourself that it's okay to have regular slips. You have a weak habit.

We could argue that some behaviors are low frequency, yet we do them out of habit. For instance, you might have a habit of sitting at your desk once every month to pay bills. You have been doing it this way for so long, it's a routine. You don't debate about whether to deal with this chore. You just do it. But no matter how routine, it's a lower frequency behavior than exercise should be and consequently not as strong. Not as strong in the sense that you probably need some cue to remind you it's bill-paying time. Maybe you have to enter it into your calendar or put a sticky on the refrigerator. In contrast, a high frequency behavior doesn't need much conscious effort to make it happen.

Frequent practice speeds learning. We could compare a low frequency when all our practice time is massed into one session with a high frequency when practice time is distributed or spaced out over many sessions with a shorter time between practice sessions. It turns out that distributed practice facilitates learning of a new ability whether it is mental or physical. A simple example is cramming for an exam. If you study for an exam more frequently over a longer period, you will learn the material better (and perform better on testing) than if you delay and spend the same amount of time crammed into the night before the test. If you are learning a new musical instrument, you will learn more quickly by practicing regularly than by spending a lot of time with it once a week. For physical recreation, some people compensate for a week of not exercising by transforming into weekend warriors who do a major bout of exercise in one day. Those persons would become more physically fit and more skilled at the sport if they spread out exercise time over more practice sessions. Why is distributed or frequent practice better?

Think of the many skills required for exercise walks in the evening. The physical skill would include adjusting gait and posture as the terrain changes from flat to hilly and maintaining balance to step over curbs and avoid obstacles. Emotionally, it's important to learn how not to be disturbed by sensations of fatigue or worries about taking time away from other responsibilities at home. Cognitively, one must learn a route around the neighborhood that is pleasing and adds up to the desired amount of walking time. Then there are practical matters to learn such as which clothes are best for the weather, which shoes are most comfortable.

All these separate skills require rehearsal and in some instances conscious problem solving until the actions are learned and memorized. The storing and recall of exercise information has a neurological basis. The more practice, the quicker those learning processes occur. Then the different systems – physical, emotional, cognitive, social start working together. Coming home to take a walk after work becomes automatic – in the door, shoes on, out the door – compared to the first couple times when it seems like a big deal. This is called procedural memory or memory for the performance of a sequence of actions. Repetition consolidates memory and waiting less time to perform the behavior again makes recall more efficient and forgetting less likely.

Frequent practice associates exercise with more situations. At the beginning it's fine to keep doing the same exercise thing, to establish one ritual and not worry about different types or ways of exercising. However, as you exercise more often eventually you will get out of your routine. By doing so you will "generalize" exercise to other environmental cues. Generalization is a process whereby a behavior becomes stronger because it transfers to or becomes associated with more situations.

Perhaps you occasionally do an exercise walk on nice weather days when you are at home with a good stretch of free time. Think of that as the original situation when your exercise walk was "learned". To make that behavior stronger you could vary the context in which you practice it. For instance, you can vary the time of day: do your exercise walk early in the morning instead of only after work. You can vary the location: do your exercise walk while out of town visiting your family. You can vary the weather: do your exercise walk on rainy days. There are innumerable cues that you can associate with your exercise walk. Some even might be subjective, such as practicing your walk when you are in a bad mood. The more situations in which you practice walking, the more cues will become associated with walking and consequently, the more your environment and state of mind will trigger the expectation to walk. The automaticity of exercise is stronger.

The reason to increase frequency of exercise to near daily is to force you to associate exercise with practically any condition. In most weeks, there are bound to be days when the weather is bad, you're not in the mood, work is demanding, or you're away from home. If you don't skip days of exercising, you are learning to associate it with the harder times not just the easier times. You learn that any day can be an exercise day. If you only exercise when everything is just right, you will have few exercise triggers in your environment and a weak behavior. (See Chapter 11 on Become Hardy to help with overcoming adversity).

Frequent practice decreases anxiety. Exercise can arouse anxiety or fear. Some examples of exercise stimuli that make people emotionally uncomfortable are: sensations of heavy breathing, wearing revealing exercise clothes in public, sweating, using unfamiliar exercise equipment, exercising outdoors, exercising at nighttime, performing exercise in a group of people, and competing with other people. If the anxiety is so strong that one feels great distress or avoids exercise in those circumstances, it approaches the level of a phobia.

The best way to overcome and "unlearn" anxiety about exercising is to gradually face the scary situation and hopefully to discover that no objective danger exists and that the stress can be managed without resorting to avoiding the situation. The elimination of anxiety, especially when a person has reacted that way for years, does not happen with just a couple therapeutic trials. If you forced yourself to walk after dusk one day, you won't necessarily cure your fear of walking in the dark. As with most learning, it's best to practice facing your anxiety provoking exercise situations repeatedly over a relatively short time period in order to stop being bothered by the situation. See the chapter on Become Hardy for details on overcoming exercise avoidance.

How Long Does It Take To Make A Habit

We can start to answer this question by looking at the precursor to a habit, namely the intention to change. The beginning of the New Year is a time of great intentions to change. But of the many people who make a New Year's resolution, about one-quarter give-up in less than a week and most by a few weeks. Clearly, the intention or mental phase does not last long enough for most people to learn a new habit.

For people who make it past the beginning attempt to change, how long does it take? Definitely more than the two weeks claimed in popular health and fitness articles. Consider the results for people studied under carefully controlled, ideal circumstances. I'm thinking of volunteers who commit to changing an uncomplicated health behavior and practice it repeatedly in exactly the same way nearly every day. Eating a piece of fruit with breakfast everyday is a good example. In the motivated person it takes about two months for that to become habit. Exercise is more complicated and takes much longer. Consider fitness centers. They lose most of their new members very quickly. Those who stay develop the habit by being consistent, working out at the fitness center a minimum of four times per week for at least a couple months. I think the magic time for an exercise to feel like a habit is closer to four months.

How do you know if you've made exercise a habit? Objective evidence of habit is showing that you regularly act the same way in certain circumstances. For example, you take an evening walk to your favorite bar every Monday, Wednesday, and Friday almost without fail. How about an animal example? Your dog always whines and acts excited whenever he sees you grab the leash and put on your walking shoes. If these behaviors are recurrent, practiced regularly for months, you safely could say they are habits.

You also know something is a habit by your inner feelings and attitudes. Not an all or nothing experience, your feeling can range from a sense of having a weak habit to having a strong habit. The stronger your habit feels, the more confident you feel and the less mental energy you need to make the behavior happen. Reflect on your habit strength with these questions. A total score of around 24 indicates moderate habit strength; 32 and above indicates strong habit strength. Re-assess yourself periodically as you progress through this program.

My Exercise Habit Strength

Rate yourself on these statements from 1-5 (1=do not agree at all, 2=agree very little, 3=agree somewhat, 4=mostly agree, 5=agree completely)	Rating
I exercise without having to consciously remember	
I exercise without thinking	
I start exercise before I realize I am doing it	
I exercise automatically	
I feel weird if I do not exercise	
I would find it hard to not exercise	
To exercise is typically me	
It would take some effort or sacrifice to not exercise	
Total score	

Figure 4.1 How strong is your habit?

Start Increasing Your Exercise Frequency

This next phase in creating an exercise habit is to gradually increase the number of days in a week that you do some physical activity.

The first couple weeks. Where to start exactly? Let's reflect on your baseline exercise frequency from the first week of self-monitoring. Is it high or low? Is this your typical frequency? Did you exercise a little more or a lot more than normal? Most importantly, did you already add an extra day or days of exercise?

If you exercised on zero days, just get one day next week. The amount of time does not matter. You could go out your door and walk for only a couple minutes to the corner. Of course you won't burn many calories and you won't have a big fitness effect. That's not important now. The important effect is more psychological, which is to go through the motions of all that is involved in an exercise outing, to start training an attitude that exercise will happen. Talking yourself into it, getting dressed, going out the door, and feeling all the feelings and thinking all the thoughts you might have. It's okay to keep your expectations low. Just moving a bit when you normally would not is a learning experience. The next time it will be easier. That's the effect of practice.

If your baseline is one day, try a second day; two days, try a third day. Again, to get that third day all you must do is something that qualifies as exercise. Time and quality are not important. If you are starting as really inactive, just one more day with a walk to the corner and back is fine to increase your frequency.

If you already added a day, don't increase again in the first week. Hold steady at that level for a bit. If you went from zero to four days all at once, it might even be better to cut back to two or three days for a while instead of risking an injury or too much stress. It's not unusual for people who haven't been exercising to jump ahead quickly. It's the equivalent of going on a crash diet in order to get results right away. The goal of this program is to create an exercise habit. Moving too fast might make you quit before habit kicks in.

The first couple months. After only a couple weeks of exercising a little more, you should feel more determined and optimistic that you will exercise. Use that momentum to add the next day and the next. Looking again at Figure 3.3, people who start at a low frequency are able to add an extra day every two weeks until they reach three days. Adding that fourth day takes a little more adjustment but is typically accomplished in two months. I emphasize four days as an initial goal in order to make exercise more frequent than non-exercise. Surely, to reach that amount you will have to exercise on some days when it's inconvenient. That's a good thing. A strong exercise habit depends on practice in different circumstances.

Avoid skipping days you scheduled to exercise and then compensating with an exercise binge on one day. You might burn as many calories had you spread out exercise over more days, but you will not make-up for the lack of practice. The point of increasing frequency is mainly to create a psychological not physical change. If all you do in the next month is go from one day with a five-minute walk to four days with five-minute walks, you're accomplishing something important.

The next couple months. Don't be discouraged if adding another day, a fifth day or sixth day is difficult. The trend of exercise change over time in Figure 3.3 shows a plateauing at four days per week. I interpret this as an adjustment period to deal with the social, psychological, and physical challenges of frequent exercise. Nonetheless, people eventually increase again somewhere between three and four months. The graph shows people fall short of six days after four months. If you have as significant physical health challenges as did these people, you may need extra time as well to reach the goal of six days. Some time to adjust to increasing exercise is appropriate. Afterward, start another effort to increase your days. Having a week of six days, then dropping back to five, and again up to six is a way to test yourself and nibble at the final target.

You are ready to increase exercise time after you have at least a couple weeks of more frequent exercise and feel comfortable with taking on a new challenge (See the next chapter on Increase Your Exercise Time). A good time to start working on the intensity and variety of exercise is when you are exercising three to four days per week (Chapters 10 and 12). Of course, if you need help with those issues now, it's fine to read those chapters now.

Exercise Often

A new habit takes much more time than a couple weeks. I hope by then you will at least be surer that you will continue to exercise. In a couple months you should feel committed to exercise and even out of sorts when you don't. Then you will be on your way to a habit.

There are other measurable features of exercise including type of exercise, length of an exercise session and its physical intensity. It's useful to modify these in and of themselves. But, the frequency of exercise is the most important predictor of an exercise habit. Stay focused on how often you exercise.

Chapter 5:
Increase Your Exercise Time

Your next assignment is to increase the number of hours in a week that you exercise. Of course, becoming more physically fit and healthy depend on putting more time into exercise. That's why we're doing this. And simultaneously, more time creates a stronger habit because new triggers for exercise are established and unhelpful, unhealthy sedentary behavior is squeezed for time and forced out.

In the last chapter on exercise frequency, the goal was to increase days of exercise per week without regard to time. Even a few minutes of physical activity practiced frequently could be effective for starting a new habit. Now is the time to increase the total amount of exercise. Using the higher standard for a healthy dose of exercise, I recommend that you eventually target six hours a week. In this chapter I will help you with some self-management tools to reach this level. It's harder to change intensity or type of exercise. Stay focused now on increasing exercise time. You can't change everything at once.

More Exercise Time Strengthens Your Habit

The beauty of increasing exercise time is that it forces you to change in other ways too. One positive effect is that you learn to associate exercise with more cues inside you and in the environment. Think about what new situations you will have to face when you exercise for a full hour nonstop as compared with ten minutes. I don't want to say a ten-minute walk is really easy, because for some people it is not. But by comparison, a long episode is more complicated.

If you're a walker and take your long walk after work you might need to walk after sunset, whereas your short walk can be done before the end of daylight. Thereafter, sunset will be another exercise cue. If you work out in a fitness center, you might have to find some kind of outdoor activity in order to not get bored by hours of indoor exercise. You might be able to dodge rain showers on a schedule of short outings, but not if you spend a lot of time recreating in the outdoors. Pretty soon it will seem reasonable and normal to go out to exercise in all kinds of situations.

Another positive effect is to have more endurance: more ability to sustain physical effort such as increased heart rate and breathing and muscular work. To have endurance, you must also learn to tolerate fatigue and to control thoughts and emotions that could make you want to stop. There is no shortcut to learning endurance. You simply make yourself do it many times until you are used to it. That is how you train yourself and how you end up not feeling burdened by exercise. Feelings like fatigue also become cues that mean exercise is okay under those circumstances.

Exercise is a time occupying activity. You might be able to squeeze in 10 minute walks now and then, but what about six hours? That much time will compete with other things and you will have to let go of some activities to exercise instead. Maybe you will gradually watch less television or give-up one of your committee meetings or be less a perfectionist about house cleaning. This is unavoidable. You will make two behavior changes at once: increase exercise and decrease sedentary, non-exercise behavior. While letting go of some pastimes can be difficult, it's an important process in creating a stronger exercise habit. (See the chapter on Prioritize Exercise.)

Start Increasing Your Exercise Time

At first, you don't have to consciously try to increase your exercise time; that should happen automatically with a higher exercise frequency. But now is when you should start deliberately working toward a much higher dose of exercise, much higher than standard public health recommendations. The Centers for Disease Control and Prevention (CDC) advises about two and one-half hours per week. Recognizing that vigorous exercise like running has extra health benefits, the CDC says if you do high intensity exercise, you only need one and one-quarter hours per week. Even lesser amounts of exercise in people who are fully sedentary will decrease risk for disease and death. Clearly, any amount of exercise at the beginning is better than none. But looking forward, in order to make exercise a habit, you cannot stop at such low amounts.

A much better goal for now is four hours per week. I recommend that intermediate step toward six hours based on what people actually do. Check Figure 3.3 again on changes in exercise over time. Even people who hardly exercise at all are usually are able to reach four hours after a couple months. For some reason that seems to be a natural resting point before exercise increases again. Later on, work toward six hours per week. That amount is associated with better health and stronger habit. Given that you probably started well below this level, you will need some plan to reach that goal. The standard self-management strategies to use for this purpose are goal setting and shaping.

Goal setting. Goal setting is a self-management strategy because a goal is a target toward which you must organize behavior to achieve. It gives you a sense of purpose so you know how much time to exercise in order to progress toward the goal. A goal gives you feedback about your performance, because you can compare yourself to the endpoint you are trying to achieve – are you close to the goal, how much exercise time is still needed this week? That comparison creates an inner tension or motivation. Once you set a goal, you don't want to fall short. You don't want to disappoint yourself or feel defeated. So, you are motivated to follow through and meet the goal. Meeting a goal gives you a sense of accomplishment and pride. Without a goal, the same exercise time would have the same physical, but not psychological effect. It's exciting to reach a goal, especially one that seems impossible. That can help make you feel excited about exercise. At the beginning when exercise is difficult, achieving a goal might be the best reward for your hard work.

A good goal is expressed in concrete and behavioral terms. "I'll try to exercise more this week" is not a good goal because it's vague and subjective. Hours per week of exercise is a perfect goal. This gives you an objective, behavioral marker against which you can compare yourself.

Shaping. Six hours per week of exercise is a long-term goal for most people. If that is far away from where you are now, how will you not feel overwhelmed and stay motivated to reach it? A problem with a long-term goal is you have to wait so long before enjoying the reward of achievement. Reward is delayed as opposed to immediate. A long delay in reward is less effective than a short delay in motivating behavior change. It would be much more effective to have a series of mini-goals so you can enjoy some satisfaction on the way to the bigger dose of exercise you are targeting. Having mini-goals also helps prevent procrastination. If the only goal you have is months away, you do not feel pressured to start changing your behavior now. A long-term goal usually requires a large change in behavior. Large changes feel overwhelming, unrealistic, scary. Mini-goals reduce big changes to smaller, realistic, achievable behavior changes.

The process of achieving a long-term goal using mini-goals is called shaping. Let's say six hours a week of exercise is what you want. To get there, break down that goal into a series of incremental steps. Each step is a closer approximation of the end point and gradually gets you to your goal. It is as if you take all the behavior required for your current amount of exercise time – and form or shape those behaviors in small steps until you have a routine of six hours. Technically, you are not shaping exercise time; you are shaping the behavior needed to put in that time. It is normal to feel overwhelmed by a goal like six hours of exercise, because most people need to make significant lifestyle changes to exercise that much. Shaping helps you break those changes down to smaller, more manageable steps.

Follow a schedule. A schedule is a plan or timetable that specifies when or how much at each interval. Look at Figure 5.1 for an example of a schedule to increase exercise gradually over four months. The increases in time are about 16 percent from week to week. This is even more gradual than what people seem to do naturally in this program (see Figure 3.3). Toward the end, you would have to add an extra half hour or more, which by then should be within your ability. At the beginning, however, you only need to add about 10 minutes of extra time in a week.

The beauty of this gradual approach is that adding a few minutes a day will help you not feel overwhelmed by the longer-term goal of an hour a day of exercise. Let's say you do four 12 minutes walks with your dog, putting you at about Week 3 on the graph. Next week, to keep making progress, you should target 58 minutes. That's only adding 2 ½ minutes to each of your dog walks. Will that feel too much an increase? Hardly. Probably the only real difficulty will be keeping your eye on the watch to make sure you meet your goal.

Speaking of using the watch, this is a good time to remind you about being accurate with your self-monitoring. A good goal involves behavior change that can be measured. Guesswork about small increments in behavior change is very ineffective in the shaping process. If all you do to prepare for your longer dog walk is say "Oh yeah, I'm supposed to walk a little longer today," how will you know if you accomplished your goal? "Longer" is too vague. Without measuring, you might walk much much further and stress yourself unnecessarily. More likely, since people tend to overestimate their exercise time, you might walk more, but probably not enough to reach your goal. So, as I warned earlier, managing your exercise behavior in terms of time will require using a watch. Be honest and stick to your goal and sooner than you think, you will be exercising a lot.

To use the exercise schedule in Figure 5.1, mark the bar on the graph that is closest to your current level of total minutes exercise per week. Write the date under the bars for each week from this point on, up to the remaining weeks on the graph. If you already exercise several hours per week and fall on the right side of the graph, make your own schedule that shows gradual increases in time, perhaps at 10 percent changes, week to week up to a week with a minimum of six hours. If you decide on another goal, calculate weekly or regular changes that will lead to it and mark your exercise graph (Figure 3.4) with your mini-goals in order to have a visual image and reminder of your plan. The example rate of change shown in Figure 5.1 is doable – it corresponds with the changes shown by real people doing this program (Figure 3.3).

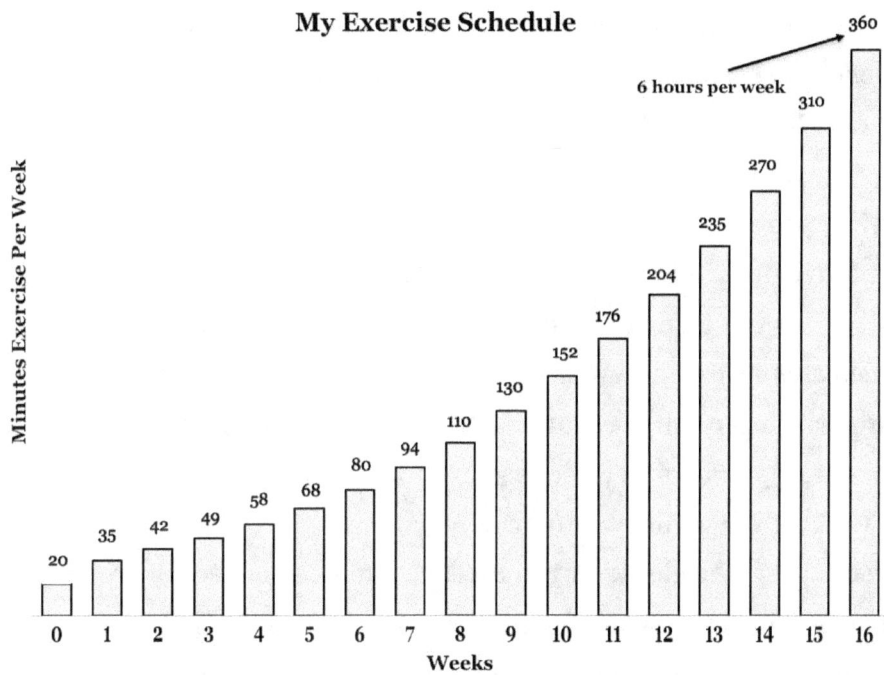

Figure 5.1 Having a goal is important to make progress and stay motivated. A large goal can be less overwhelming if broken down into smaller, gradual steps.

Before beginning the next week, calculate the extra time needed to make your weekly goal. You have options for how to distribute the extra time. If you have not reached four days per week, you could achieve two positive results at once by putting the extra time in a fourth day of exercise. If you are still adjusting to a higher frequency of exercise, like four days, split the extra time evenly among days. This makes the time increase less impactful. After reading the chapter on Vary Your Exercise Intensity, hopefully you will be inspired to work on having an endurance day or one long bout of exercise each week. You could add all of the time increase to just one of your workouts to build endurance. Exactly one hour per day is often not possible and not as beneficial as mixing up the length of workouts.

Self-Monitoring Recommendations

Recording exercise time. Write your exercise time along with type of exercise in the same graph and diary or equivalent as shown before (Figures 3.2 and 3.4). Time yourself, don't estimate.

If you take breaks during a workout or want to measure small increases in time, there are more accurate alternatives to a clock or stopwatch. Try an electronic activity monitor, fitness tracker, smart phone app, indoor aerobic machine, or bicycle computer. These stop the clock when you stop moving. Some will give you feedback about your speed, the elevation you ascended and descended, the route you took, and calories you burned. When your workout is uploaded to a computer or smart phone, you might be able to see graphs or tables of various exercise results including comparisons with previous times for the same walking or riding route. If that information ramps up your enthusiasm, great. Use self-monitoring as a motivator.

Aside from these nice features, the most important measure right now is time, not speed, calories, climbing etc. Stay focused on increasing time and frequency without worrying about speed. When you are regularly exercising four days a week, you're ready to work on quality of exercise – see the chapters on varying intensity and type of exercise for that issue. Moreover, regarding all the nice ways your exercise data can be displayed in computer and smart phone apps, the one result that needs to be recorded in a graph, is total exercise time for the week. Continue with the weekly time and frequency graph you started at the beginning.

Monitoring steps. Some activity trackers give you a cumulative total of your steps and time moving during the day. Some also can notify you if you haven't moved or have been sedentary for a certain amount of time. These devices can encourage more walking and less sitting time, but be aware of the following issues.

If you have a problem being too sedentary (See chapter on Prioritize Exercise) an activity tracker that measures time not-moving can help you reduce sitting time simply by the motivating effects of self-monitoring. Although I will encourage you to become less sedentary, I will not ask you to measure it so that your diary will not be too burdensome. No worry, if you don't measure sitting time, you should feel confident about decreasing it simply by eliminating some sedentary behavior. If you eliminated watching TV as soon as you arrive home, your physical activity or moving time probably would go up.

If worn all day, activity trackers include any steps and activities of daily living, not just intentional walking or exercise. You need to distinguish between the two because the harder behavior to develop is exercise for exercise sake. Only exercise goes in your record, so an activity monitor would need to be used to record those episodes separately.

Setting a goal for number of steps can be a great motivator, but what goal exactly? A common one with no health or scientific basis is 10,000 steps. Not only does that include non-exercise behavior, but also 10,000 steps is not much higher than the equivalent of the insufficient public health (CDC) recommendation for exercise. In fact, it turns out that risk for serious health problems is reduced most by people who exceed 15,000 steps per day.

Weighing yourself. Body weight might be a good addition to your diary, but it's absolutely optional. If you hope exercise will help you lose weight, it's important to start seeing both results so you can learn about their relationship – how much and what type of exercise produces a weight loss. Seeing that weight loss on the scale and in your log is a reward and consequently will increase the likelihood you'll repeat that exercise.

I have a couple recommendations about weighing yourself. Use a consistent method – upon awakening, undressed, after toileting, before eating and on the same scale will give more accurate and reliable results. Like recording exercise, you should record your weight, whether or not you like the number. It will not help you to understand the exercise – weight correlation if you omit days you think you gained weight. Finally, record at least once a week. There's nothing inherently unhealthy or damaging about weighing yourself even daily. It's a number that you can use dispassionately to manage exercise behavior.

Changes In Fitness With More Exercise Time

What a difference it makes to increase exercise time! Look at the example of an exerciser who followed the gradual schedule toward a total of six hours of walking per week (Figure 5.2). Not only is our exerciser's time increasing, but the amount of calories he or she burns from exercise increases too. Considering this person's weight of 240 pounds, he or she is losing about a pound a week upon reaching the goal of six hours. The chart also assumes that our walker is becoming stronger and able to walk faster over time as he or she accommodates to exercise.

	time exercising per week	calories burned
Week 1, walking at 2.5 miles per hour (24 minute miles)	35 minutes	191
About week 4 to 5	60 minutes (1 hr)	327
About week 8 to 9, walking at 3.0 miles per hour (20 minute miles)	120 minutes (2 hrs)	764
About week 12	180 min. (3 hrs)	1145
About week 13 to 14	240 min. (4 hrs)	1527
Week 16, walking at 3.5 miles per hour (17 minute miles)	360 min. (6 hrs)	2618

Figure 5.2 An example of the improvement in fitness and calorie expenditure as a 240 pound person progresses toward a large amount of exercise

Be careful to not compensate for exercise by resting more. Some people end up being less active around the house after a good workout. Let's face it. If you're tired from a long walk, it can be tempting to recover by lounging around. This compensation can be really subtle. For example, people who are encouraged to use standing positions more at work, unconsciously compensate by sitting more at home. Biologically, people may have a built-in need or tolerable limit for a total quantity of activity. When that is reached, unconsciously we want to rest. But too much sedentary time and sitting especially, predict poor health independently of how much one exercises. So, the best strategy is to add exercise time and to maintain the rest of your physical routine as normally as possible.

Be careful to not compensate for exercise by eating more. You might think you need to eat something to recover. How about a sports drink? Yes, food is important after a certain amount of exercise. But if you have a 100-calorie energy drink after running or walking just one mile, you will have consumed the calories you burned. Exercise can be an excuse to indulge. It's best to stick to your regular meal pattern and not use exercise as snack time.

Exercise Is A Healthy Preoccupation

Although lots of exercise is physically healthy, some people mistakenly see it as weird. In my former field of research, eating disorders, some articles appeared in which the authors asserted that a lot of exercise could be a psychological disorder. They gave the example of male runners who log 50 miles a week of running and claimed they might suffer from a male form of anorexia nervosa. Supposedly, instead of being obsessed with food, they are obsessed with exercise, they are self-centered and trying to compensate for an inner defect and they are as pathologically concerned about being as thin as are female anorexics.

But I knew from my experience with a group of racers who spent 15 hours a week on the bike that we might have been obsessed with training and our weight, but it felt healthy and fun, not pathologic. So, one of my research students and I conducted a study to test this exercise disorder idea. It turned out that high mileage male and female runners indeed wanted to stay thin, they felt concerned even guilty if they missed workouts, and running took away a lot of time from other things in their lives. But, compared to women diagnosed with an eating disorder who were dysfunctional on every measure, the runners were not depressed or anxious, they felt satisfied with their physical appearance, they did not feel guilty about eating, and they had positive self-esteem. In other words, they were well adjusted.

I told you this story because in our society where dedicated exercisers constitute a small minority, it's easy to see them as deviant in a negative way. It's also easy to feel intimidated by the idea of joining them, which is why some people put down exercisers. The reality is, people actually feel better psychologically, have a better body image, and manage stress better when they exercise a lot.

Having said this, if you are exercising so much that you are hurting your work or relationships or causing physical or medical problems, it's time to re-evaluate. See Chapters 9 and 12 for ideas on including other people in your exercise and responding to negative social feedback. Chapter 10 deals with when it's good to cut back on exercise in order to stay healthy and how to cope with that.

Increase Exercise Time

If you're serious about improving your fitness and making exercise a strong habit, it truly is necessary to build up the time you put into it. You cannot have both, a casual sporadic schedule of exercise and real fitness. Make a goal for increasing exercise time and work toward it in small, but steady steps. Achieving goals inspires even more behavior change. In the long run, an exercise habit becomes stronger when given a lot of time because more situations become associated with it.

Chapter 6:
Prioritize Exercise

Lack of time is the most common excuse for not exercising. Indeed, exercise is a time occupying activity and the problem is how to add it to a busy schedule. It turns out that people spend as much time now as decades ago working, shopping, doing house chores and taking care of other people. And leisure time remains steady at about five hours per weekday, more on weekends and just slightly less for working adults with children at home. The difference is not that people are busier; rather, leisure time has become more sedentary. People spend more time reading, socializing, watching television, and using electronic entertainment and less time than before being physically active.

To create time you must re-order your daily activities and get your workout before you spend all your time doing less important things. To have a strong exercise habit, you must make it a priority. A priority is not just something you think is important, but something so important that you are sure to do it before other things. To prioritize is an action word and means doing things in order of importance. This chapter presents the psychology of prioritizing and how you can use this self-management strategy to create time for exercise.

Ineffective Prioritizing

"After I open my mail, check my messages, and start dinner, I'll go for my walk." "I'll feel a lot better about taking time for the fitness center if I get some more work done." "First I am going to do everything else. Then, if I have time left, I'll exercise."

This kind of planning is a setup for skipping exercise. If you put all the familiar time demands first, the daily chores and duties that you already do habitually without a fight, they probably will take all the time you have available, including time you hoped to save for exercise.

If you are struggling to exercise, subconsciously, you may even intentionally allow just enough time for those other chores so it's too late to exercise. That will give you an acceptable excuse to procrastinate and reschedule your walk for another day. Putting exercise way down the list of things to do can be an avoidance strategy.

If you save exercise for last because it's not fun, you probably are putting more rewarding daily activities first. Even opening the mail or doing housework may be more rewarding than exercise. This contingency puts rewards first rather than using rewards as a motivating consequence. The best way to train a new behavior is to provide a reward after its performance.

"I can't exercise today, because I have my ..... book club, cooking club, wine club, bible club, gun club, quilting club, speakers club, needlework, artwork, wood work, newspaper puzzles, internet games, fundraiser meeting, PTA meeting, neighborhood meeting, museum docent meeting, animal shelter meeting, student mentor meeting, library board meeting, TV watching, video watching, sports watching, picnicking, entertaining, and relaxing." You cannot prioritize too many pastimes over exercise and still be able to create a physically active lifestyle. Something has to go if you plan to reach that goal of six hours per week of exercise.

Effective Prioritizing

Effective prioritizing can be summed up by the formula, "First I will do my exercise, then I will _____ (do all those things less important than exercise)."

I used to follow this strategy on weekends with my cycling club.

We scheduled rides at 6:30 am in order to complete our workout early, before we were consumed by family obligations. Usually my family was just getting-up when I returned home from the bike ride. They didn't miss me and I didn't have to pull myself away from anything later in the day to exercise.

Early morning hours at fitness centers are busy because people learn they are more likely to stick with exercise if they do it first thing in the day, before work. Early morning exercise is one of the safest schedules for an exercise habit because everything else is prioritized lower. There is no temptation to surrender time to other things, because they are avoided completely until after exercise.

Clearly, family isn't less a priority in the sense of importance than exercise. Neither is work. But I already am naturally inclined to be with the family and to work, whereas sometimes I have to force myself to exercise to get that out of the way. Exercise must be urgent, pressing, high on the list simply because it is so tempting to avoid. Therefore, prioritizing can also mean doing things in order of difficulty. Getting exercise first is a form of discipline that works because you delay gratification and comfort until you have done the more difficult thing - your workout. One of Grandma's Rule sums this up as "Work first, play later." Later, when exercise truly is fun, you can still prioritize it, but then enjoy a little word reversal: "Play first, work later."

Become Good At Prioritizing

Learn the best timing for exercise. Although a great self-control strategy, exercise early in the day is not always practical or desirable. All that you must do to prioritize effectively, is make exercise happen before any activity that predicts, causes, triggers, sabotages, or leads to not following through with planned exercise. Learn from your patterns of helpful and unhelpful sequences of activities. Be patient, it may take some time to learn from trial and error when exercise must be scheduled ahead of other behaviors. Facilitate your learning by writing a list of such experiences. See Figure 6.1 for an example.

What happened first	What happened next, what I learned
Opened my mail. Got distracted by some bills I didn't expect.	Spent time checking my records instead of going on my walk. It's hard to resist the mail. I do better with exercise if I deal with the mail later in the evening.
Had a hard day. Thought I'd relax on the couch before hitting the gym.	Really sleepy. Skipped the gym for today. It would be better to relax after exercising. Maybe exercising would energize me and I wouldn't need to waste time on the couch.
Went home first to check on the kids before meeting friend for a hike.	Too many demands from the kids to leave home. Next time, I'll leave better instructions for the kids so they can make do without me until I finish hiking.
A new project assigned to me at work.	Went to the fitness center as planned. Felt more energetic to start on the project. Probably would have wasted time feeling resentful if I skipped exercise.
It's my turn to clean the house.	Knew I better swim first, because once I start cleaning, I always find more work that needs to be done.
A full day of appointments. Went to the early yoga class first.	Too risky to wait for the night class. My meetings might run late or I might feel too tired.

Figure 6.1 Describe experiences when exercise was prioritized or not and what happened after.

In these examples, opening the mail, relaxing on the couch, and checking on the kids were antecedents or triggers for not exercising. Good prioritizing would be to avoid getting involved with these activities until you finished your planned exercise. But considerable self-control might be needed to delay these deeply engrained behaviors. Sometimes, the best strategy is to physically avoid the tempting situation altogether, such as don't even touch the mail until you finished your walk. Don't even look at the couch or even go home before you do your exercise.

Reward exercise with lower priorities. Putting exercise first gives you the opportunity to create some rewarding consequence. Save something you especially enjoy or something that by comparison to your workout will be easy or pleasurable. If taking a shower, relaxing, spending time with the family, accomplishing something at work are positive experiences and saved until you have done a good bout of exercise, they act as rewards for exercise. That contingency increases the probability of exercise. You look forward to exercise because it is followed by positive experiences. Thank goodness, because while you're trying to become a regular exerciser, you want all the pleasurable consequences you can find to outweigh the negative sensations and side effects of exercising.

If you don't know which activities might be good rewards to schedule after exercise, don't worry. Any high frequency activity is a candidate for prioritizing below exercise. A high frequency activity would be something you do habitually every day. Reading your messages, responding to notifications on your smart phone, calling your boyfriend, and neatening the house. None of these might seem like positive rewards for exercise. But because you do them all the time, there is a history of rewarding consequences that have made them strong, engrained behaviors. Exercise is a low frequency behavior that needs motivating consequences. Opening your mail is a high frequency behavior that you feel compelled to do daily. Refraining from doing it until you get your workout provides a reward. See the chapter, Reward Yourself for Exercising for more help with this self-management skill.

Become more time efficient. The real reason people save exercise for last is that they simply do not want to exercise. The excuse is, exercising first will upset the schedule - there won't be enough time left to take care of other important obligations. Let's test that prediction, that saving some activities until you finished exercising will take too much time away from other obligations. What would happen as you embark on your exercise outing? Exercising first would create some tension to get it over with so you can go ahead with other things. That's exactly what you want; a motivating force – the anticipation of getting back to your daily chores – to urge you to complete the bout of exercise.

Take advantage of that tension. Tell yourself, "I have to exercise so I can go home and get ready for dinner." Then, assuming you now feel squeezed for time because you delayed your responsibilities, you probably would be more speedy and efficient and able to accomplish what you predicted would be impossible in less time.

I'm thinking of another rule, Parkinson's Law that says work expands to fill the time available for its accomplishment. The challenge is to allow enough time for exercise and other things, and to have confidence that when squeezed for time, you will be strongly motivated to finish all those chores you delayed for your exercise. If it's any reassurance, as you become more healthy and fit, you will be able to do more things in a fixed amount of time because you will move faster, lift and carry weight more easily, and feel less tired by activity.

Don't talk yourself into procrastinating. Listen to your self-talk, the stream of thoughts running through your mind as you approach the time to exercise. If you catch yourself starting to say you can wait to later, you could be in trouble. Talking about procrastinating leads to procrastinating. Interrupt that temptation with some alternative, more helpful self-talk that emphasizes how important it is to exercise. Practice self-talk that says exercise is a priority and then get out the door for your walk before that other voice disrupts your exercise plan. Any self-talk that tells you to delay or skip exercise should be a cue to immediately drop what you are doing and exercise first before you let avoidance take over. See the next chapter on Clean-up Your Self-Talk to learn more about this important self-management skill.

In the meantime, here are some examples of self-talk that prioritize exercise, especially when you are facing choices.

"If I'm going to become more fit, then I have to do this."

"Either I'm serious or not about my physical fitness."

"This IS important to me."

"I have to do this. This is my job."

"If I wait until later, I won't feel like it. I better exercise now."

"I better get out the door now before I start doing other things."

"I'm thinking about skipping my workout because I'm feeling lazy. That's not a good enough reason."

"Either I do nothing today or I exercise so I can get off medication."

"What's more important, my health or doing that?"

"What's worse, having to do this exercise or having heart bypass surgery?"

"If I don't do my exercise, then I won't be around to do those other things anyway."

"My exercise is more important than spending time doing crafts."

"I know people don't like when I take off to walk, but if I don't, I won't be good for anybody anyway."

"I can't do everything. Something has to go if I am serious about getting healthy."

"I can't expect other people to understand. I have to do this for me."

"People will have to learn to function without me."

"I feel guilty taking the time for exercise, but I'm doing something for myself. I'm taking care of myself. That feels good."

Let Go Of Sedentary Activities

People who exercise a lot eventually create time for it by cutting back on things that do not contribute to their fitness. The simplest method is to reduce the number of meetings you attend, organizations you belong to, volunteer services you give, and time spent doing hobbies, socializing and entertaining in physically inactive ways. Sometimes total abstinence from an activity is easier than moderation. For instance, cutting back on hours of daytime TV watching on the weekends still exposes you to TV watching and temptation, whereas total abstinence says TV is not an option. You end up not even thinking about it. The fewer time obligations and distractions, the less struggle to make room for exercise. Dropping sedentary pastimes is difficult and requires some psychological adjustment over time.

You can think of it as a kind of grieving process. Let's say you enjoy watching TV sports on the weekend more than you should. You've been told you need to exercise for medical reasons. At first you might deny that you have a problem. Then denial turns to anger that you have diabetes and have to start exercising. When the reality hits that you must change, you might feel sad about missing your sports shows. You might imagine that life won't be as much fun. However, as time goes on spending more time being physically active, you realize that you can live without some of those less healthy pastimes. The active you is the new normal. You no longer feel a sense of loss.

There is no shortcut to letting go. You simply start by changing your schedule and hopefully discover it's not as hard as you expected.

Spend Less Time Sitting Down

It's possible to spend a lot of time exercising <u>and</u> a lot of time being sedentary. As one goes up, the other does not necessarily go down. In fact, people can defeat the benefit of more exercise by using that as an excuse to be less active the rest of the time. So, being physically active and inactive are not necessarily correlated with each; they are independent behaviors. And it turns out that they are independent health wise; a lot of down time predicts poor health even in exercisers.

What is sedentary? It implies passive, low energy activity. But now a public health definition is emerging that specifies sedentary behavior as sitting (or lying down when not sleeping). That's because sitting is the worst offender for health. Too much sitting predicts disease and faster aging in adults. According to this definition, standing and driving, for instance, are not considered sedentary. Standing burns twice as many calories and for the sake of health, is preferable to doing the same activity seated.

Too much time on the bottom is probably the most common health risk factor today. Most people including young people spend more than half of their waking hours sitting. An effect of modern living, sitting has become more extensive than time spent sleeping. Sitting time only increases in older age. Sitting too much is especially a problem in the workplace. Rarely do employed people reach a healthy amount of moving time or number of steps at work. Not surprisingly, people tend to be sitting deniers. Even the most active workers like hospital nurses overestimate how much time they are moving as opposed to sitting.

Sit less. Think about being off your bottom for a couple hours more per day. How? Stand more. Stand up at your desk every so often. Stand during commercial breaks on TV. Stand and move when you are talking on the phone. Avoid continuous sitting for more than an hour without a standing, moving break. Use a reminder from a fitness app or timer on your phone or computer to stand and move. It's not enough to exercise an hour and then sit on your bottom for 23 hours. Work on both, exercise and sitting time.

Increase Your Exercise By Making It A Priority

Most people struggle with exercise because they act like work, chores and everything else are mandatory, whereas exercise is optional. If you are serious about improving your health and fitness, exercise no longer can be an option. It must be mandatory. And to help make it happen, prioritize it. Take control of your schedule and exercise before or instead of less important, easier, or more ordinary activities whenever possible. Spending a lot of time doing other things first is risky, because you might lose your motivation. Making exercise a priority gives you good feelings of satisfaction and accomplishment that help you to accept letting go of sedentary activities. We are not too tired at the end of the day because we get too much exercise. We are tired because we do not get enough.

Chapter 7:
Clean-up Your Self-Talk

Exercise is enough of a struggle already. It will not help to repeatedly tell yourself "This is too hard," "I don't have enough time," "I feel like I'm going to die," or "I can't wait for this to be over." How well you stick to your exercise plan, how much you enjoy it, and how competent you feel depend greatly on what you say to yourself. Self-talk is the force inside the head that pushes you in one direction or another, especially when facing challenging exercise situations.

Positive changes in self-talk will occur automatically if you follow my recommendations for increasing the frequency and amount of exercise. But it is best to take stock of your self-talk now and to speed the process of mental change by deliberately practicing alternative thoughts that will help you to stick to your goals. This chapter will help you learn to recognize thinking patterns during exercise and how to modify them to your advantage.

The Nature Of Self-Talk

It helps to have a good attitude about exercising. "Exercise is fun." "I like to exercise." Surely if you think this way, you will have less trouble increasing exercise than if your attitude is "Exercise is a drag." But a good exercise attitude doesn't come easily. Attitudes are general outlooks on life that take time to form. If you are having trouble, you might have a long history of negative ideas about exercise and now those old ideas have resurfaced. Besides their persistence, another problem with old attitudes is that you can't see or hear them. Attitude is not observable, not concrete. In fact, technically, attitude is a concept designed by psychologists to represent a hidden mental process that governs behavior without our knowing it.

If you want to have a better outlook on exercise, you need to begin by changing your self-talk. Self-talk is the private conversation inside your head. It is the conscious, concrete and immediate manifestation of the more complex mental concept, attitude. Because self-talk is concrete and observable, you have the power to deliberately change it. Changes in self-talk will translate into changes in attitudes and beliefs over time. But most importantly, changing self-talk will have an immediate effect on changing behavior. Unhelpful, self-defeating self-talk about exercise makes you avoid and give-up on your exercise plans. Helpful, self-enhancing self-talk makes exercise more pleasurable and more likely to happen.

If you focus your awareness on your thinking, you can hear yourself talk silently. You don't have to make yourself think or invent thoughts. There is usually a steady stream of thoughts that are spontaneous and can be brought into awareness simply by paying attention to them. But once you focus your awareness on thinking, your thoughts or self-talk begin to change because unconsciously you want to direct them one way or another. It's like breathing. You breathe automatically, but you can control your breathing if you focus your attention on it. You control your thoughts by silently and intentionally saying other thoughts that alter, embellish, or replace the spontaneous ones. Learning to increase exercise will depend on these two skills, awareness and control of self-talk.

Assessing Your Self-Talk

It's easy to hear yourself thinking, but if you want to have a better attitude about exercise, you need to write down those thoughts. Systematic recording of self-talk will force you to be honest about your thinking and how it affects your decisions to exercise. After you identify your typical thoughts especially when you're struggling with exercise, you'll be ready to create more helpful self-talk.

Many self-help books on health behavior change provide a questionnaire or list of positive and negative thoughts. The reader can simply check the relevant ones and use the questionnaire to start practicing new thoughts. But these are thoughts or attitudes written by the author and not necessarily the exact ones that affect you. I will help by giving you tips on keeping a good self-talk diary, but I will not give you the answers. Only you know the unique and personal ideas inside your head that cause you to exercise. It takes time to keep a diary, but it is a powerful way to change your behavior.

The Self-Talk Diary. Start your diary and don't stop until you find a pattern or good examples of helpful and unhelpful talk. It's best to record some thoughts during every exercise episode rather than skip around. The diary should be a list with three columns like Figure 7.1, the situation, your self-talk, and the consequence of your thinking.

Under "situation", write about the context of your self-talk. What was the situation? What was happening? This is the antecedent or trigger for the self-talk that follows. After a while of keeping a diary, you will learn the situations that typically lead to helpful or unhelpful self-talk. Check Figure 7.1 for examples.

You might simply write the exercise, like example #2 "Walking uphill". Or write some detail about the situation if it might be relevant to your self-talk, such as #5: "Walking the recreation path. Lots of people dressed in exercise clothes, looking fit." You will want to remember that being around fit looking people is the context or trigger for feeling self-conscious about your appearance. Example #6, "Riding my bike. It's hilly. Pedaling hard" turns out to be a trigger at first for thoughts of powerlessness. Thinking in anticipation of exercise can be crucial for whether you follow through with your plan (#10). Feelings and sensations can be a context for exercising, such as "...feeling tired" (#1), "Feeling down..." (#8), or "Breathing really hard" (#9).

"My self-talk" – write what you were thinking or saying to yourself. If you don't spontaneously hear thoughts, talk to yourself. Ask, "What am I thinking?" It's likely that whatever you say will reflect your current feelings. Write your exact words. If you call yourself a wimp, go ahead and write it. Though you might not like seeing your words on paper, you will be better able to change those than the self-talk you try to forget.

The examples of self-talk in Figure 7.1 cover common thinking problems in struggling exercisers. Most essentially are thoughts that it's hard, I don't want to do this, I can't do this, or I feel bad. Preoccupation with unpleasant physical sensations, e.g., sweating (#4), fears of injury (#9), and thinking I look bad (#5) also are not infrequent. Example #3 is worrying about time pressure, which is a typical trigger for quitting. Another common problem is minimizing the importance of exercise, such as example #7. All or nothing thinking, like example #8, usually involves telling yourself to skip exercise because you already have blown-it and skipped other days – this is a frequent self-defeating rationale for giving-up. All these are typical ways people talk themselves out of exercising. There are innumerable variations. The challenge is for you to find your own. Use these examples to sensitize you to thinking traps you might fall into.

Hopefully you already have some helpful, encouraging self-talk to counter negative thoughts. Be sure to write those thoughts as well. Examples #6 and 7 show self-talk that corrected the negative thoughts. Writing these thoughts can help you identify arguments you have with yourself. Was the negative thought followed by something more helpful or vice versa? In the column for "consequence", you will have an opportunity to see whether answers to negative self-talk with something positive or at least neutral, led to a good outcome.

"Consequence." Write what happened after the self-talk. You should focus on consequences for your exercise. The example diary shows some typical consequences that might occur, such as whether you finish the exercise episode or quit early, whether you do the hard workout or skip that for the easier one, whether you have a reasonably positive experience or feel bad physically or emotionally. Notice in some examples, the person stated some intention to do a certain activity and subsequently did or did not. That type of sequence could be especially useful to record. At this point, you should have some plan or goal for most of your exercise sessions. Becoming aware of self-talk and how it affects completing your plan will help you identify and correct unhelpful self-talk.

The term consequence implies that whatever happened was the effect of the way you were thinking. However, you cannot be sure which thoughts or self-talk "caused" the next event or which event was the consequence of the preceding thoughts. You can't prove causation when it comes to mental activity, but at least you can identify a chain of events. First something happens, then you say something to yourself, and then something else happens. In example #3, maybe the exerciser cut his walk short because he was bored and worried about doing other things. Or maybe the real reason was the long walk felt too hard and boredom was just his excuse to stop. Regardless, example #3 is a good chain of events or sequence for this person to remember. The next time he is doing a hard workout, thinking about boredom is a warning sign that he might quit, no matter the real reason. Later you will learn that when you don't know exactly why you do something, you can control that behavior by breaking the chain of events that leads to it (See the chapter Cue Your Exercise). The self-talk diary is a record of a chain of events that includes a mental behavior (self-talk is behavior, just verbal and sub-vocal) and some event that follows it.

Tips on recording self-talk. Record every day for a while, long enough to have a good sample of self-talk during different types of exercise conditions. Conditions can differ according to intensity of exercise, weather, time demands, mood, physical well-being and energy, and so forth. Your motivation to exercise and your exercise experience can be very situation specific and consequently different conditions might trigger different self-talk. For example, you might have a good state of mind when taking a leisurely walk around the neighborhood, but become negative when you try a more ambitious walk up hills. The idea is to accumulate some examples of self-talk when exercise is easy and when it is difficult, psychologically or physically. Having a list of positive self-talk will be useful in the future when you need to answer negative thoughts with more helpful alternatives. Having a list of unhelpful self-talk will make you alert to triggers for stopping or avoiding exercise.

Thought recording is tricky because there is a steady stream of thoughts once you pay attention. Which thoughts do you write? Thoughts that occur spontaneously without forcing yourself to think and which discourage or encourage you to exercise are worth recording. If you are not sure, write the main thoughts that repeat themselves. Thinking about the flowers as you walk might not seem to be important self-talk, but maybe later you will discover that helps to keep your mind off boredom and to keep walking. If you are not hearing any thoughts, you could ask yourself, "What am I thinking now." Answers to that question are a legitimate reflection of your attitude.

Try to get below the surface. Self-talk can be superficial and a shorter way to say something more complex and relevant. Imagine you are thinking, "This is not easy." Is that telling you much? Why is it not easy? So, what if it is not easy; why might that concern you? If below the surface you have an exaggerated worry, "I might have a heart attack" (example #9), you probably identified a thought that is more relevant to your urge to quit. Ask yourself a question about your thoughts to dig a little deeper. An easy question to ask is, "And what else am I thinking at this moment?" If you think, "This is a long time to walk" and you question yourself, maybe you'll hear an answer such as example #3, "It's getting boring. I have a lot of work to do today." Boredom and worry about work are common obstacles to exercise. Detecting those thoughts will help prepare you to counter them with helpful self-talk.

It is harder to admit, especially in writing, negative thoughts that reflect on you as a person, your ability or personality, such as "I can't do this." Consequently, there is a tendency to deny those, whereas negative thoughts about circumstances external to you are easier to admit. Examples #4 and #5 concern unpleasant exercise experiences, but embarrassment about physical appearance is the more sensitive one. It takes some courage to be honest and write such thoughts in a diary.

When you self-monitor, you become more attentive to the behavior and that attention can trigger changes in behavior, usually in the positive direction. People don't want to think negatively, so keeping a diary of thoughts might inspire you to start changing, even before you understand what type of thinking makes a difference for your exercise. Like overestimating exercise and underestimating eating, there is an unconscious bias toward emphasizing your positive thoughts. It is okay to put a positive spin on the situation, but at least write the negative thoughts too. Seeing both will give you some record of the helpful thoughts that you end up using to offset the more automatic unhelpful or negative thoughts.

Finally, mentally rehearse or repeat the main thoughts you are having so you can remember to record them right after exercise. Write down your self-talk as soon as possible after your exercise. Try to avoid waiting until later in the day. Thoughts are not like time on a stopwatch. They are more subject to distortion and forgetting. A way to eliminate the problem of memory is to record thoughts immediately with a voice memo app on your smartphone.

Keeping this record does not mean you don't have to keep an exercise record. Combine the two if you want, but exercise needs to be recorded everyday indefinitely.

What was the situation? What was happening?	My self-talk: What was I thinking or saying to myself?	Consequence: How did that affect me, my feelings, what I did in that situation?
1. Getting ready for my walk, feeling tired	I really don't want to do this now	Decided to walk tomorrow instead
2. Walking uphill	This is really hard. I think I'm too tired to walk uphill. Preoccupied with how bad I feel	I turned around and walked a flat route
3. Trying to do a long walk	This is a long time to walk. It's getting boring. I have a lot of work to do today.	Cut my walk short. Felt guilty.
4. It's hot. I'm really sweating	Can't stand sweating. This is disgusting.	Felt really uncomfortable. Didn't enjoy my exercise today
5. Walking the recreation path. Lots of people dressed in exercise clothes, looking fit	Feel like I look stupid and out of shape. Feel embarrassed Feel awkward, weird.	Tried not looking at people so I wouldn't feel self-conscious. Then got off the path & walked elsewhere

6. Riding my bike. It's hilly. Pedaling hard	I can't do this. Just concentrate on pedaling. Stay focused on the top of the hill. I can make it	Super tired at the top, but I made it
7. Am supposed to do a longer walk today.	This isn't that important. Who needs long walks. But a long walk will increase my endurance. It's worth it.	Walked 60 minutes, my longest ever. Yippee!
8. Feeling down	Not in the mood to exercise today. What the heck. I skipped yesterday so might as well skip today.	No exercise today ☹
9. Breathing really hard.	This is not easy. I might have a heart attack.	Stopped & rested
10. On my way home from work. I have a ton of things to do.	I wonder if I'll have enough time to exercise. I don't have a choice. I have to stick to my exercise schedule	Exercised first, then did other things

Figure 7.1 A record of your Self-Talk should include the situation, your self-talk or thoughts at the time, and the consequence or events that followed.

Make Your Self-Talk More Helpful

Helpful and unhelpful self-talk. Unhelpful self-talk is any type of thinking that makes you avoid exercise, quit early, exercise badly, or exaggerate unpleasant physical or psychological experiences. Because the strength of an exercise habit depends on a consistent high frequency, most troublesome is self-talk that makes you skip a planned exercise episode. Helpful self-talk keeps you focused on your goal, encourages you to follow-through with your intention, and makes you feel good.

When I started mountain bike racing, I worried too much about riding off narrow trails to hazards on the sides, like riding over a steep drop-off or riding into trees close to the trail. It seemed, the more I worried about riding into an obstacle, the more my bike wanted to move in that direction. Sometimes my fear was confirmed. I saw a threat off-trail and ran right into it because I was so focused on it. When I asked more experienced racers how they avoided hazards and stayed on-trail, they said, "Look where you want to go, not where you don't want to go."

This advice can be understood literally and figuratively. Literally, turning your head in the wrong direction will force your body there as well. Golfers, tennis players, skiers, motorcyclists and sports enthusiasts of all types learn to look in the direction where they want the ball or their body to go, because, as the saying goes, "the body follows the head." Figuratively, dwelling on negative self-talk will turn your behavior in the wrong direction. Behavior follows the mind. You can talk yourself into thinking or doing things that are not to your advantage. So, "look (or talk) where you want to go, not where you don't want to go." This is the motto of positive self-talk.

Develop alternative, helpful self-talk. What can you say to yourself the next time you are in a troublesome exercise situation that will be more helpful? Think of alternatives that counter the unwanted thoughts, correct them, emphasize a positive side, or simply distract yourself. Make your new self-talk realistic. If you feel too tired when walking strenuously, you do not have to say, "This is easy, I'm a super strong walker." Your alternative self-talk should be reasonably believable, maybe not 100 percent believable, but enough so you can say it with some conviction, so it doesn't seem completely phony. Your alternative self-talk does not even need to be positive. Neutral is fine, just not negative.

Work on your self-talk on the go, as you experience trouble during exercise episodes and on paper in your self-talk record. An example of a new form to write alternative self-talk is shown in Figure 7.2. New statements in writing will make them more real. You will have a record of helpful things to say that you can rehearse at home, outside the stress of an exercise crisis.

Situation	My self-talk	Consequence	Alternative, helpful self-talk

Figure 7.2 Write alternative, more helpful self-talk to practice the next time you face a difficult exercise situation.

Examples of helpful self-talk and thought control. Although the exact words you use must be your own, there are different methods to correct or control your thoughts (Figure 7.3). Use a way that best fits the situation.

Method	Example
Self-instruction: Telling or reminding yourself what to do.	You are walking a hill, feeling tired and thinking of turning back home. You say, "Concentrate on making it to the top of the hill. Walk strong, head up."
Self-efficacy messages: Positive statements about your ability to do something, about yourself as a person or your accomplishments.	You are trying to do a long walk, but getting bored and wondering if you are able to walk so far. You say, "This is a long time to walk, but I can do it. I'm a lot stronger than I used to be. There's no reason I can't handle this."
Rational self-talk: Statements designed to correct self-defeating or false thinking by responding with a more correct or logical self-statement.	You overate snacking before going on your walk and thought, "What's the difference, I already feel like a slug, it doesn't matter now whether I walk or not. You respond by saying, "I <u>will</u> feel better if I walk, even though I might be sluggish...and it <u>does</u> matter – I'll still burn calories and I'll learn not to skip exercise."
Reframing: Translating your interpretation of an experience into words that are more helpful, comforting, and adaptive.	You're walking uphill, breathing really hard and your legs are feeling heavy. You are thinking, "I feel so tired, this hurts." You

	translate those feelings into, "I can feel my muscles working, I'm getting a really good workout. This is good for me."
Imagery: Concentrating on a mental image that bolsters your confidence or performance.	You're walking with other people. You are starting to fall behind and want to catch-up. You concentrate on your arm and leg rhythm and think of yourself as a machine, like a locomotive, moving fast and strong.
Rehearsal: Preparing for an encounter with a troubling situation by warning yourself how you might feel and how you will act.	You worked late and you want to get your walk in, but you know you'll be tired and will be tempted to skip it and go to the kitchen instead. You say, "No, I'm not going to do that. I'm going straight to the bedroom for my walking shoes". And then you mentally rehearse passing the kitchen for your walking shoes.
Distraction: Repeating a word or short phrase to override or distract you from other thoughts.	You are riding your bike into a headwind, breathing hard. You find yourself dwelling on how long and tiring it is. Instead, you start counting breaths, "One, two, three ...twenty," then count from the beginning again

	over and over.
Thought stopping: Interrupting thinking by telling yourself to stop.	You worry the family will be upset with you for taking a walk before dinner. Rationally, you know they won't, but you are obsessing anyway with guilty thoughts. You say, "Stop!" loudly inside your head and repeat, "Stop!" after each guilty thought until they disappear.
Acceptance: Telling yourself it's okay to not be perfect or to be unskilled at something.	You started an aerobics class and are having trouble learning the routines. You think, "I'm such a klutz. Maybe I don't belong here." You counter that by saying, "It's okay. I am a little klutzy now and a beginner. That doesn't mean I don't have a right to be here. I'm here to save my life, not to impress people."

Figure 7.3 Try different types of alternative thinking and thought control.

Trouble shooting tips. Be alert to troubles overcoming negative self-talk. Try these solutions.

1. "But my negative thoughts are true." It's normal to not fight thoughts that seem true rather than distorted or irrational. For instance, the new exerciser keeps telling herself, "I am so out of shape," as she tries to keep up with her aerobics class. Okay, maybe she is out

of shape, but is it helpful for her to dwell on that? Can she think of some alternative that also is true, but supports her effort, such as, "I might be out of shape, but I'm here and I'll get better." Self-talk should be judged by its effect, not just its validity.

Sometimes just saying the true but unflattering thought using a kinder, accepting voice is enough to interrupt any negative effect.

2. Difficulty thinking of positive self-talk in the moment. Try writing a list of useful self-statements ahead of time. Rehearse them at home when you are not in the middle of an exercise challenge. Rehearse them with some feeling. Imagine yourself repeating that self-talk in situations when you might be at risk for unhelpful thoughts. You also could record self-statements in a voice memo app on your smartphone and play them as needed during your workout.

3. Can't think or talk to myself when I'm exercising strenuously. Intense physical effort takes a lot of attention and can interfere with speaking in sentences (even silently). Try a distraction technique, like simply repeating a word or phrase that will not involve much mental effort. I found counting breaths when cycling up a hard climb was all I could think, but that kept me from thinking about being tired. Listening to music helps to mask negative thoughts.

4. Negative thoughts keep surfacing even though I'm practicing positive self-talk. Negative thoughts are overlearned mental reactions. Rather than stress when a negative one intrudes, don't try to analyze why you still have that thought or whether it's right or wrong. Just let yourself hear it and then let it go. Use that thought to immediately cue you to resume repeating your new helpful talk. Negative self-talk should be a reminder to stay focused on helpful thoughts.

5. I don't believe what I'm saying. Choose alternative thoughts that are reasonably believable, maybe even neutral at best. Reasonably

believable means the thought is not absurd; rather it is possible and correct to some degree. Imagine a scale of believability. If you tell yourself "I can't do this" and the alternative "I can do this" is only ten percent believable, that's enough to start. Just because the thought is not 100 percent believable, does not mean it is untrue. Repeat your new self-talk and refrain from analyzing whether it's true. Just repeat it. The more practice, the more natural and believable the alternative thoughts will be.

6. Am I just thinking of excuses? An excuse is a face saving justification for skipping exercise. A reason is the actual cause or explanation. It is better to admit the real reason, so you can address it with alternative thinking. Let's say the real reason you feel like quitting is you feel weak and out of shape, but your excuse is, you are busy. Trying to talk yourself out of being busy probably won't motivate you to keep going. Ask yourself, "Am I just making an excuse?" Often just admitting to making an excuse is enough to stop that thought.

Changing Behavior Also Leads To Changed Thoughts

Positive self-talk encourages you to keep exercising and to reach new levels of fitness and enjoyment. Don't be discouraged if after practicing the strategies in this chapter you still are repeating negative self-talk that brings you down. Developing believable alternative thoughts can be difficult. Making them automatic takes practice.

The point of cleaning up your self-talk is that changing thinking leads to changed behavior. It might be reassuring, however, to know that sometimes change goes in the opposite order. You have to change your behavior before you start talking to yourself differently. Just go through the motions of exercising, follow an exercise schedule, increase the number of days on which you exercise and the time will come when those old negative reactions are easier to control and will disappear.

Chapter 8:
Cue Your Exercise

An exercise cue is a signal or reminder to exercise. Any stimulus in the environment or inside the person can become a cue if it is paired with exercise repeatedly over time. This is called conditioning. Because it can be so difficult to make yourself start a session of exercise, the conditioned cues that are most helpful to recognize or create are those that precede or coincide with exercise. Cues or circumstances that lead to giving up planned exercise work against you and need to be identified as well. You can become more aware of exercise cues and then consciously manage them to your advantage.

When establishing a new behavior, it is helpful to intentionally create cues to remind you of the behavior that needs to be performed. What do you do when you are to take a prescription medicine? Do you rely on memory? Probably not. Most people use the medicine bottle as a visible reminder to take a dose, like putting the bottle out in the open on the bathroom or kitchen counter. Using a pill sorter that separates the doses for a day into little compartments is visual feedback for following the schedule. Posting a chart. Putting a sticky on the refrigerator that says "medicine". These are ways we stimulate a necessary response that is new and maybe unnatural. If you are organized and use reminders, it's easier to follow a schedule. The new behavior you are trying to learn starts becoming more automatic.

The Conditioning Process

It's a sunny morning. You are looking at your calendar and see a 10:00 am meeting with a friend to walk the recreation path. Out of the corner of your eye, you notice your walking shoes by the front door.

Your water bottle is on the kitchen counter. It's time to get ready for your walk.

All these are cues to prepare for an exercise walk. Any one of them would be a good reminder – seeing your 10:00 am meeting to walk, certainly would. The mental image of your friend waiting would be too. But so would the others. Just the sight of your walking shoes should remind you of an exercise appointment. Maybe you have a history of taking walks on sunny mornings. It would be hard to single out one cue as the strongest, most motivating reminder. Together they form a background for the act of preparing for exercise. After some history of this context being associated with your morning walk, any one or combination of cues will become a learned reminder that automatically drives you out the door. It's like a ritual. One thing is associated with another and leads eventually to the desired response – exercise.

One reason people struggle at the beginning is they have no exercise rituals, no routine or sequence of cues that put the process in motion. They're still on the learning curve. Consequently, it's normal to be disorganized and haphazard and to wonder when, how will I get my workout this week? If you are beginning with a very low frequency, like trying to exercise on just one or two days a week, learning exercise cues will be a slow process, because you only have a couple conditioning trials each week. Be patient. Just force yourself to go through the motions – exercise. Exercise does not occur in isolation. There will be environmental or other cues in the background. As you increase your exercise frequency, the associated cues that make you follow-through with your exercise plan will become stronger and more motivating. In the meantime, you can speed up the process by becoming more aware of your exercise cues and intentionally creating some other reminders and rituals.

The importance of cues for health behavior like exercise is easy to recognize in eating. People are biologically programmed to eat when hungry; learning is not required to stimulate eating. However, exactly when and where eating takes place is learned by pairing environmental cues with the pleasure of ingestion. If you snack standing at the kitchen counter or in front of TV, those cues can trigger appetite. If you have a routine of taking candy from your office mate's desk, the sight of her desk will stimulate a craving for candy. One way people learn to control unwanted eating is to eliminate food cues whenever possible. Not eating outside of a normal dining place and keeping unwanted foods out of the house are classic ways to control appetite. Out of sight, out of mind.

With exercise, however, you need to develop the opposite strategy. Instead of reducing triggering cues, you need to keep exercise cues in sight and in mind so as to increase the probability of exercise. Any stimulus that increases the likelihood you will exercise is an exercise cue.

What Are Your Exercise Cues?

In case you are thinking, "Gee, I don't have any exercise cues;" you're wrong. You have at least one important cue already – your exercise diary. This is a visual reminder that exercise is supposed to happen and hopefully will inspire you to get moving so you will have something to enter on the diary. An exercise diary is more than assessment; it causes behavior change too because it is a cue to exercise.

In addition to your regular exercise diary, for a week or few weeks, write something about the situations leading up to your exercise episodes. Record the circumstances around each one long enough to be clear on the cues associated with you getting ready to exercise (See

Figure 8.1). If you think you already know your exercise cues, do the self-assessment anyway. Not all exercise cues are in our conscious awareness. Environmental stimuli that you think are irrelevant might actually be signals if they have been associated repeatedly with exercise. For example, your walking shoes are within sight on the floor. Although you already know exercise is on your schedule, seeing your shoes reminds you to get ready, even though you are not consciously aware of reacting to the sight of your shoes. The best assessment at this point is increase your awareness and to record as much as possible about the situation. Practically anything in the environment, external or internal, could go on your chart. To help jog your awareness, I made columns to write typical contextual cues. Start by filling in a couple of your exercise cue situations in Figure 8.1. If you think other circumstances determine whether you will or will not exercise, make a form of your own to record those as well. Check the examples.

What pattern do you see in your exercise cues? Do you typically exercise at a certain time of day? Have you created some reminder cue like a note on your calendar? Are you more likely to exercise when it's sunny and warm? Are your exercise episodes always after housecleaning? Do you have belongings around the house that trigger thoughts of exercise? Are there any cues that regularly precede an exercise episode?

Time of day	Weather	Location	What is happening? Whom am I with? What is my mood? How am I feeling?	What is making me think of exercise, reminding me to get ready?
8:45 am		My desk in the den	Reading the news. Checked my calendar.	I see a full schedule later in the day. Better get my workout soon before it's too late.
6:00 am		Kitchen counter	Updating my exercise diary	I see I need one more hour to make four hours this week
6:00 pm	Light rain	Just walked in the house	Feeling harried, not happy about the weather	My rain shell and waterproof shoes are in front of my closet. I put them there last night to make sure I didn't ignore the fact I'm supposed to exercise tonight

11 am	Nice	Office at work. Papers on the desk.	Mindful of the time. My friend sends me her usual text asking me to walk with her during lunch	Her text is a great motivator to follow through with my walk

Figure 8.1 Recording exercise cues or reminders will help you create stronger exercise rituals

Cue Your Exercise

Calendar your exercise time. The most common exercise cue people create is an exercise appointment written in a personal organizer such as a calendar or weekly planner. If you already organize your week in writing, why not take advantage of that system and make an appointment with yourself to exercise?

I like the tone of that expression – an appointment with yourself. Too many people who struggle with exercise do not make self-care a priority. To make an appointment with yourself is an act of self-respect and commitment. If you have a calendar full of appointments taking care of other people, how about creating a time slot for yourself? You'll probably be better able to take care of everyone else if you do.

How far along are you in terms of increasing exercise time and frequency? You should have a plan for the week. You should know what you intend to accomplish. If not, go back to the chapters on increasing exercise and write a schedule of mini-goals toward the big goal of six days and six hours. You should not be scheduling exercise episodes in your calendar without a sense of purpose.

Now write your schedule for all the bouts of exercise you need to do this week. Do not write one day at a time. Commit yourself in advance. If you need to get five days and four hours, but only put one day in your calendar, aren't you taking a risk that the other days will be filled with appointments? You wouldn't wait to the last minute to write an appointment for the dentist. Why should exercise be left to chance? The point of a calendar is to have everything written in advance, so you can organize your time and stay focused. Exercise must become as important as anything else that deserves space in your calendar.

If you keep an appointment calendar, you probably don't need to be told – put it in the open where you can see it or on an electronic device you use regularly! Or use a phone app that notifies or reminds you of the scheduled workout. Yes, seeing impending exercise appointments will keep you focused and prepared.

Be careful of being over ambitious. Don't fill in every day on the calendar with exercise if you are not at the level of regular exercise. Only schedule enough to meet your goal for maintaining or increasing your frequency.

Only schedule times you are confident you will meet. To make written exercise appointments a meaningful cue, they must be paired with the behavior you want to stimulate - follow-through with exercise. If you blow-off an appointment, entries in your diary will not become a cue. Only stimuli that routinely precede the desired behavior are conditioned cues. Don't ruin the potential of an appointment calendar for behavior management by being too undependable. If you are not sure you will have the time to exercise, don't write anything. Otherwise write your appointment and stick with it, no matter how hard it might be. The next time, keeping an appointment will be less difficult because now you have some history of the diary, indeed, being an antecedent to exercise.

The power of regular exercise times. If you calendar the same exercise times week after week, eventually those times become a powerful cue. You don't even need the written entry in a calendar. My cycling friends and I have a regular group ride early Wednesday mornings, year-round. I don't have to think, "Will I or won't I?" or "When today will I?" It's automatic. Wednesday morning is committed and protected. The person who has no regular schedule is faced with more decision-making and consequently more opportunity to procrastinate, forget, or surrender time to other types of appointments. Having a standard time removes competing options. Over time, 8:30 am became my group ride. There is no longer any argument about that time slot. I say "No" to appointments for 8:30 am, because it is already reserved – it's my golden hour, my exercise, self-care, and social time.

Developing fixed times may not be best for everyone or every exercise episode. It's good to be flexible. Nonetheless, I recommend you commit to at least one regular time slot per week. At the beginning, it is good to have a repetitive routine and ritual. With practice, there is a good probability of following through without much resistance from yourself or others. Psychologically, it's strengthens your commitment. It's concrete practice with prioritizing exercise, with being assertive and declining other requests for your time.

Make use of other exercise cues. What else reminds you to exercise? How about these: walking shoes, gym bag, heart rate monitor, energy bars, water bottle, MP3 player, fitness magazines, gym pass, dumbbells, exercise rubber bands, yoga mat, exercise DVD, bicycle, sun hat, fishing rod, golf bag, Lycra shorts, swim goggles. All these say "exercise". Visual cues such as these can become powerful stimuli to get ready for your exercise outing. Put them where you can see them.

People who are trying to lose weight learn to hide tempting food cues and avoid places where they might be exposed to unwanted food. For exercise, try the opposite. Get those exercise stimuli out of hiding and strategically place them to encourage you to exercise. If you have to search through the closet to find the walking shoes, you are much less likely to use them than if they are by the front door, visible the moment you enter the house.

Some fitness trackers can be set to notify you if you are behind in meeting a goal for activity. Take advantage of technical gadgets that might remind you to move. But if you use one, follow-through with the reminder, otherwise that cue will not be an exercise cue. Effective cues are reliably paired with the desired behavior.

Control Cues That Make You Skip Exercise

The best intention to exercise can be undermined by unexpected, compelling circumstances. You must accept these times. But if there are recurring situations that make you give-up, you should identify the chain of events leading up to them. Where are you? What is happening around you? What exactly made you decide to forgo exercise? In the previous chapter on "Clean-up Your Self-Talk," you might have discovered typical thoughts that make you quit. Now, identify the concrete cues or stimuli in the environment that precede quitting. These are high-risk situations. Figure 8.2 has examples of triggers for skipping exercise. Add some of your own in the blanks and make your own form to record details of times that you skipped planned exercise.

One reason I developed a habit of doing my training bike rides early in the morning, even on cold Vermont days, was because entering my office building turned out to be a cue to skip my ride. I remember when my strategy was to work for a couple hours while the temperatures warmed and then to head out on the bike. The problem was, once I walked in the building, there were students and colleagues who wanted to talk, there were letters and emails I felt compelled to answer, and there were unfinished lectures on my desk. It took great effort to break away from these pressures and not surprising, often I failed. I learned that the sight of unfinished work and working colleagues were not stimuli for getting on the bike, they were stimuli for getting on my desk chair. My solution was to stay away from work cues before doing my morning ride. First, I tried entering the building, still in Lycra cycling clothes, just to drop-off my backpack before continuing on my ride. Even that exposed me to temptation to quit. Ultimately, I learned to leave my backpack in my friend's car in the parking lot so I wouldn't have to see anyone or my desk inside the building. Out of sight, out of mind. That might seem like a gimmick, but it worked for me.

I was fortunate to have the flexibility of a university professor's schedule that allowed me to mix-up bouts of work and exercise as I pleased. But as my wife liked to say, "Unlike you, most people have 'real' jobs and can't exercise during the day." So true. And how many people face exercise killer situations like a house full of demanding children and family when returning home. If you can resist these pressures, if you can be assertive and tell people to wait, if you can shore-up your resolve with inspiring self-talk – great. But if you need extra help, try stimulus control. Like many of my clients did, don't walk into the house until you have gotten your exercise episode. Stop at the fitness center on the way home. Take your walking shoes to work and do your walk before heading home. I had one client who kept her walking shoes at the back door in the garage. After getting out of the car, she would change shoes and walk the neighborhood before entering the house.

Taking control of cues to exercise or not exercise can be similar to the process of prioritizing exercise. When you prioritize exercise, you organize behavior in a sequence so that it occurs before other high frequency, compelling obligations and activities. In the case of controlling cues, you might avoid cues or delay exposure to cues that are associated with competing activities and skipping exercise, such as being at home or work at certain times.

There are a couple examples in Figure 8.2 that call for problem solving, not just avoidance. If you have a lot of visitors that conflict with your normal exercise schedule, perhaps you could do something active with your visitors that works for you too. If feeling fat or having a new hairdo routinely limits exercise, it would be best to face those situations and learn to cope in some way other than skipping exercise altogether. The psychology of facing challenging or high-risk situations is examined further in the chapters on Become Hardy and Don't Give Up Your Exercise.

Time of day	Weather	Location	What is happening? Whom am I with? What is my mood? How am I feeling?	What is making me think of not exercising, led to skipping exercise?
Midday	Cool	Employee lounge	Anxious to get out of the building to go on my run	Co-workers talking to me about a project deadline.
Saturday morning	Great weather	Home	Disappointed I can't go on my normal group ride this morning.	Friends visiting from out of town.
After work	Humid. Might drizzle	On way home	Planned on running in the park, but had my hair done today.	Worried that my new doo will be wrecked exercising tonight
7 am		Bathroom	My weight went up. Feeling fat.	No way I'm going to aerobics today feeling like this.

Time of day	Weather	Location	What is happening? Whom am I with? What is my mood? How am I feeling?	What is making me think of not exercising, led to skipping exercise?

Figure 8.2 Record the cues or stimuli associated with times you skip exercise.

Vary Your Exercise Cues

Repetition of an exercise ritual is helpful at the beginning in order to have a sense of routine, to have fewer decisions to make, to think less about when and where exercise will happen. Going regularly to the 6:00 pm aerobics class, scheduling weekday walks during lunch and a golf game Saturday morning without fail, doing sit-ups before bed every night. These routines will trigger exercise without a lot of thought.

Even better is when you expand the variety of circumstances for exercise so you are not limited to just one ritual. Let's say the 6:00 pm fitness center class is your original learning situation for exercise. The time and place you went from zero exercise to two, three, four days a week with exercise. That schedule is predictable and feels comfortable. If you now added a morning walk, you would learn to associate exercise with a whole new set of cues: different environment, different clothes, and different time.

Another suggestion is pick a time of day or day of week when you are least active. Perhaps you are totally inactive in the evening at home. That time slot represents an entire collection of cues to be sedentary. If you inserted physical activity into that time slot and stuck with it, over time evening would have a whole new usefulness. And you would solve two problems at once: decreasing cues to be sedentary and increasing cues to exercise. Find a new time to make an exercise time.

Cue Control Works

When people fail to change their exercise, they tend to blame their weak wills. But behavior isn't just a matter of self-control. Exercise does not occur in a vacuum. It's triggered automatically by environmental cues that remind us and stimulate us to get moving. How automatic does your exercise feel now? Answer the questions in Figure 4.1 on habit again to see if yours is becoming stronger.

We can increase the probability of following through with exercise by creating a routine that associates exercise with specific reminders and cues. After achieving a reasonable, regular dose of exercise, it's time to add more exercise cues to your repertoire. Learning to associate exercise with a variety of circumstances makes the behavior stronger and more deeply engrained.

Chapter 9:
Encourage People to Support Your Exercise

Starting an exercise habit is an act of self-care and making you a priority. But chances are someone else will benefit too as you become more physically fit. Functioning better with other people actually is an important reason for many people to exercise more. They want to participate more fully in the family, to keep up with their active friends, to stay healthy for the grandchildren, to accomplish more at work, to inspire their partner to exercise more too. Although your exercise might help other people, receiving the support you need might be a challenge. Are other people welcoming and encouraging your exercise? Or are they unsupportive or even trying to sabotage your effort?

Taking time away from other people can be a major stress and some sensitivity, negotiation and assertiveness are required to get family and friends on your side. Becoming healthier is a good thing, but can affect the status quo with other people. Success with changing health behavior, such as improving nutrition and losing weight, quitting smoking, and exercising more, is determined to some extent by social relationships and help from others. If support does not come naturally in your social environment, there are ways you can encourage people to be a help, not a hurt.

The Nature of Social Support

Social network and help. One concept of social support is about the size of your social network or quantity of relationships, the depth of relationships, and how often you interact with other people. Being surrounded by people who are positive and care about you and best of all, share your interest in being physically active, will encourage your exercise habit. Having a large or small social network is influenced by opportunity such as having a job that exposes you to a lot of people. Personality also determines social network. People who are more extraverted tend to have more active social lives. As you can imagine, changing these factors, opportunity and personality, is not easy. In principle, the larger the social network, the better. But simple quantity is less important than having at least someone who supports your exercise.

The other concept of social support is the type and amount of help you receive from other people. People can support exercise by giving tangible help. Examples are: gifts and money for things like exercise gear or a fitness center membership; other people helping with childcare or housework in order to free time for you to exercise; friends who want to walk with you to encourage your new habit. Information or advice is a type of support, such as instruction from a friend on how to ride your new bike or tips from a walking partner on dressing for rainy weather. Emotional support refers to things that people do that make you feel cared for, that bolster your feelings of self-worth, that encourage you and help you to talk over a problem. In other words, anything people do that gives you a "Go for it", "We approve" message about your exercise.

Unsupportive people. Unsupportive people don't offer practical help or emotional support. Instead of accepting your need for time to exercise, unsupportive family members do not cooperate with changes to the home routine. Unsupportive workmates intrude on your exercise break. Unsupportive people criticize and complain that your exercise time is taking time away from them. Other kinds of guilt trips are common, like complaints of feeling left out and complaints of not being able to keep-up with your exercise. Forcing social events and sedentary pastimes on you when you are trying to make a more active lifestyle is a problem. Accusing you of being too obsessed with exercise is unhelpful. One way or another, unsupportive people do not collaborate on your exercise. They do not welcome and celebrate the new you.

Why? The most forgiving explanation is that people sometimes do not understand how hard it is to make yourself exercise. They don't understand why you must stick to a schedule, why you must make other changes in your lifestyle, why you need to exercise so much. They might not even buy into the idea that increasing your exercise is important for your health. Being unsupportive is not necessarily malicious.

If the number one excuse for not exercising is lack of time, probably the leading excuse for your partner not helping is that your exercise takes time away from him or her. It's an inconvenience. If you are always talking about how you need to get moving on exercise, other people might not believe you will do it this time; they might not take you seriously. Your improving fitness and self-esteem can upset the status quo in a relationship. Maybe someone feels threatened – what are the implications of your new lifestyle for him or her? Will becoming more healthy, functional and self-confident affect your role in the relationship? Maybe someone who has his or her own fitness problem is jealous that you are succeeding. Their lack of support is an external projection of their own feelings of failure. Sadly, sometimes people don't want their loved one to get better. The bottom line is, instead of seeing things from your point of view, unsupportive people may be reacting in their own self-interest.

Changes in exercise and social support over the lifespan. Generally, physical activity starts dropping off by the time people are in their thirties. That's when making it in the work world consumes a lot more time and becomes a priority over recreation. Single people maintain exercise better than married people. And young married people with children decrease exercise the most. Therefore, social support for exercise is all the more important for partners who have extra time demands and extra domestic responsibilities.

Not surprisingly, spouses and partners influence each other's exercise. Over time, physical activity in couples becomes more similar, especially during older adulthood. If one partner drops off, the other partner's exercise will too. And the reverse is true. A physically unfit partner is more likely to increase activity if his or her partner exercises a lot. If both partners in a relationship are inactive, starting an exercise program together is more effective than doing it individually.

Reflect on Your Social Support

Hopefully this discussion has made you think about social support you are or are not receiving. Instead of giving you any more leading suggestions by questioning you with a checklist of social support, how about writing your own answers using the open-ended questions in Figure 9.1. Try to be specific. Instead of writing vague descriptions such as, "I like it when my husband shows he cares". Give concrete examples such as, "I like it when my husband tells me he is proud of my weight training." Don't hold back. Be honest and say what you really think about how encouraged you feel by other people.

My Support for Exercise from Other People

1. How open are you to other people about your exercise program? What are you open about and to whom are you open? Are there some things that you are not telling others? If you are open, why? If not, why are you not more open with people?

2. What do people do that helps you with your exercise? What do they do that doesn't help or you don't like? Write the names of several people: family, friends, workmates, or others. Answer the questions for each person.

3. What can you do to encourage people around you to be more helpful or supportive? Write something specific for each person. If you need more people to support your exercise, who would that be? What kind of support are you missing? What ideas do you have to add such people to your social support network?

Figure 9.1 Write about the encouragement you are or are not receiving from people.

Increase Your Social Support

Support is an interaction. People can't support your exercise if they don't know you're trying to do something. Are you telling everyone, telling people on a need-to-know basis, or keeping it a secret? Some people are comfortable sharing or asking for help. Others are reluctant to broadcast changes in their personal health behavior.

If you're like most people, past attempts to exercise haven't lasted very long, so you may be reluctant to make a public announcement. You may not want to get your own hopes up, let alone the hopes of others until you have accomplished something. The purpose behind exercising more might relate to some emotionally charged issue, such as body image or needing to lose weight. Many people do not want to draw attention to these issues and consequently avoid talking about any form of weight control behavior. Modest people can worry that talking about self-improvement will be taken the wrong way, as boasting rather than reaching out for encouragement.

Openness and self-disclosure are personality traits and not easy to change. Therefore, the best way to seek help is what comes naturally. Nonetheless, it is good to be flexible. If sticking to your exercise schedule is at risk, you may need to reach out for support even if this is uncomfortable. If your commitment is wavering, it will help to speak to other people even if that feels risky. Public statements about needing to exercise will strengthen your intention to follow-through. When someone is getting in your way, you will need to make clear how important your exercise is and stick up for your rights.

Be assertive. My bicycle racing friends and I would talk a lot about how our training regimens and time away from home on the weekends to race were being accepted by our families, in particular, by our spouses. How to balance home life and the huge time commitment of an athletic career was a major challenge. And I learned there was no one correct way to negotiate. Some guys and gals on our team would propose to their partners a schedule of races and training days they wanted to do during the season and essentially ask for permission. Usually this led to cutting back on cycling commitments. In contrast, other friends had a non-negotiable attitude and did not invite objections from other people; they followed a schedule that was best for their racing career.

No matter how these discussions are handled, if you are serious about developing a substantial exercise habit, other people will need to understand and support you. The likelihood of a positive reception depends on how you communicate your needs. Here is a simple formula for what to say:

Your intention or desire

Why it is important for you

What help you might need

What benefit there might be for the other person

Empathy for any undesirable impact on him or her

For example:

"Honey, I need to do my morning spin class before we go to your mother's house. I know you're anxious to leave. But if I exercise first, I'll be in a better mood and feel more energetic to visit your mother. I'm trying to be consistent with 5 days a week of exercise and can't skip today if I'm going to stick to that schedule. Thanks for your understanding."

Trouble-shooting assertiveness. Being assertive is not easy for everyone. The term "assertiveness" was popularized in psychology by therapists who specialized in communication skills and couples relationships. It represents a healthy midpoint between passivity and aggression. People who are passive are afraid to speak their minds and let other people infringe on their rights. Aggressive people force their desires on people without respecting the other person's feelings. One style can drive the other. A common pattern is being too passive and suppressing feelings and desires until it's intolerable, then blowing up in anger. Assertiveness is supposed to be a solution to these extremes.

Assertiveness begins with an honest statement to your partner, friend, colleague, whomever regarding your exercise. Use the formula above. Say what you need to do while also being sensitive and appreciative. The emphasis must be on honesty; honesty with yourself and with the other person. If you pretend it really doesn't matter if you skip a planned exercise episode, you won't advance and you risk the rebound toward aggression. Get outside your comfort zone if need be and follow through with your intention.

Being assertive requires that you believe your requests are reasonable, that you have a right to exercise, that it's normal and healthy to take time for yourself. People who have trouble being assertive doubt themselves too much. They sacrifice their own interests to please the other person, even if that means sacrificing basic needs like self-care and health.

Fear is an obstacle to being assertive. People avoid assertiveness because they fear their partner will feel angry, manipulated, hurt or unappreciated. If they push ahead with their own needs, some people imagine, they will feel guilty. Which is worse, skipping exercise and remaining in a state of bad health or feeling guilty? Too often, the answer is the latter.

If you avoid being assertive, a good way to feel more comfortable is to go through the motions, to start acting assertive and see what happens. The consequences will probably be more positive than the reaction you fear. Before asserting yourself, question your reluctance with this formula: "If I assert myself (by saying or doing something), _____ will happen (the other person will act or do, I will feel)." For example, "If I tell my husband 'I'm going to my spinning class this morning before we leave,' he will get angry and accuse me of not caring about his mother." Okay, that's your prediction about the dreaded reaction from him. And what prediction about your own reaction do you make? "I'll feel terrible and his hurt feelings will ruin my day."

This scenario is a hypothesis or guess – I say guess, because having been unassertive, you don't have much experience to know what will actually happen. Testing your hypothesis hopefully will result in one of two outcomes: either the reaction from your partner isn't as unsupportive as you imagined or you are better able to handle the negative reaction than you imagined.

Comfort with assertiveness comes from gradual learning that the feared consequences of standing up for your rights, sticking to your exercise plans, asking for support and so forth are manageable. If you have a history of not being assertive and not making your self-care a priority, it will take some time for other people to learn that you are serious this time. This learning comes with experience. There is no shortcut.

Other communication techniques. Here are a few ways to strengthen your communication and encourage other people to listen.

The "Broken Record". You assertively stated your need to exercise or asked for help. You're confident you are being reasonable, fair and not asking for too much. But the other person refused or tried to argue with you. What do you do now? Like a broken record – as in an old vinyl recording – or maybe a scratched CD that skips and repeats itself, you simply repeat your assertion. Repeat it as often as you need for the person to understand you are serious and that you will not back down. Below is an example:

The key to the Broken Record is to not debate or argue with the person and to not respond to guilt trips. Deflect those attacks by agreeing to the extent appropriate or ignoring them and repeat your assertion. It may take a few times for the person to realize you aren't going to play the game and that you intend to do what you want. It might seem heartless or antagonizing to repeat yourself, but at the beginning, if you have a history of being unassertive, you must train your partner to understand you won't back down and surrender your rights. Eventually, your partner will be more accepting and cooperative.

the Broken Record	
You	**Him**
"I want to hike with the nature club Saturday morning. Would you please cover the kids for a couple hours?"	"Do you really have to hike? We have a lot to do this weekend. It seems like all you're doing is exercising."
"Yes. I want to hike with the club for a couple hours."	"But you already have hiked this week. Isn't it time for you to be with the family!"
"Yes, but I want to hike with the club for a couple hours."	"Well, how do you expect to be gone when the kids have to get ready for soccer?"
"I'll be hiking with the club and would like you to cover the kids while I'm gone."	"Don't you care how this affects us around here?"
"Of course. But I'll be gone for a couple hours hiking."	"Okay, but I'm not happy about this."

"I-statements". The opposite, "you-statements", begin with the word "You" followed by some description of the person that generally is received as an accusation: "You don't care that I'm trying to exercise more." You-statements usually are not objective descriptions of behavior, rather interpretations: "You don't care..." Because you-

statements can be taken as attacks on character, they make the person more focused on defending him or herself instead of helping you solve your concern.

When you state your concern with an "I-statement", you begin by saying how you feel or what you experience. "I feel stressed by trying to stick with this exercise program." The focus is on you. You take responsibility for your feelings and you don't blame the other person. You are being open and sharing your experience without saying it's their fault. Which kind of statement is your partner more likely to listen to?

You-statement	Translated into I-statement
"You don't help me or care about me trying to lose weight."	"I feel discouraged trying to lose weight and need help."
"You never give me the time I need to go to the gym."	"I need 3 mornings a week at the gym."
"I'm exercising now, but you're not doing anything. You should worry about your health too!"	"I would really enjoy exercising with you sometime."
"You act so hurt when I leave for my exercise class, like you don't want me to take time for myself."	"As much as I need to stick with my exercise, it's hard for me too when I take time away from us."

Agree with the other person. When facing resistance to your exercise, find something your partner says that you can agree with. The normal inclination is to defend yourself and try to negate the other person's objections. If you put up a wall and won't listen to any feedback that conflicts with your exercise, the other person probably will become less supportive, maybe even hostile. At least be a good listener and acknowledge any reasonable complaints. It's okay for people to disagree with you or to disapprove. Just because the other person doesn't support your exercise or has a legitimate objection, doesn't mean skipping exercise is the only solution. If you let the other person talk and listen to the feedback, the tension over your exercise might be defused. That _is_ a solution.

Agree with the other person	
Your partner	**You**
1. "The money you're spending on a personal trainer is adding up. We can't afford to go to concerts every week like we used to."	"You're right. That cost is cutting into other things. I miss some of the concerts too."
"Does that mean you're willing to give up the trainer?"	"No, but I understand what you're saying about the expense affecting us."
"It seems like the people you run with are mostly women. I'd feel more comfortable if you did your running with other guys."	"You're right. It turns out there are a lot of women runners in this group."
"Well, what about running with guys instead?"	"I know you'd feel more comfortable with an all-guys group. For now, I'm sticking with these people – it's working for me."

Your partner	You
2. "You're so obsessed with exercise now; we're not socializing as much as we used to. We're losing our friends because you only want to do outdoorsy things with people."	"I see that. My lifestyle is becoming more physically active and I'm gravitating toward friends who share that interest. And this is affecting you too."

Praise people who support you. If you have helpful friends and loved ones who are proud of you and do something nice to support your exercise, it's easy to be appreciative. But if people who are not helping surround you, you cannot simply command them to be supportive. You will need to teach them to be gradually more supportive by expressing appreciation at every opportunity.

Unsupportive people will not suddenly buy you a fitness center membership. So, you will have to find small steps, any small gestures toward caring about you and your exercise so you can start teaching them to be helpful and considerate. Truly unhelpful people might not do a single thing that makes it easy or pleasant to exercise. So, you will have to find something that at least approximates being helpful, even if it is coupled with unhelpful behavior. If you're careful in how you express appreciation and follow the examples, most likely your partner will feel appreciated and will start acting more supportive.

Verbal praise is an excellent form of reward because most people like positive social attention and will work to get it. Moreover, verbal praise is an effective teaching technique, because you can clearly specify the desirable behavior in concrete terms. That will make it easier for the person to repeat the behavior.

Verbal praise for helpful support
1. Label the behavior you want to encourage in clear, concrete terms
"You hiking with me helped a lot. I had to hike faster than normal. It was a good workout. Thanks."
"I really appreciate you telling me to go to aerobics class when I felt like skipping it. I needed that push."
2. Show appreciation when your partner makes small steps toward being supportive. Ignore the unhelpful behavior and give positive attention for the helpful.
You asked your husband to take your old treadmill out of storage and set it up in the recreation room. He grumbled that he was busy, but finally brought it to the room. Although he didn't move it exactly in place and connect the power as you would have liked, he did make some effort to help. You said: "Thanks so much for getting that into the house. There's no way I could have done it myself."
You invited yourself to hike with some friends although you worried about keeping up with them. They walked much faster uphill than you and left you behind. You felt lonely and disappointed they abandoned you. At the top of the hill, they were waiting and you said, "Thanks for waiting for me. I like walking with the group. Maybe I can keep up with you for a while on the downhill."
You're excited that you set a new record for a long walk and told your boyfriend all about going non-stop for one and one-half hours. He didn't look-up from texting on his phone, but he grunted an acknowledgement. You said, "I can't help but feel proud of myself and at least you listened. Thanks."

Quality time with others. I had a client who enjoyed short walks in the evening with his wife, but he also did a long solo hike every Saturday. His goal was to summit all 4,000 foot peaks in the Adirondacks in up-state New York. Having started overweight and essentially sedentary, he was excited about his growing fitness and learned that he needed at least one long endurance episode each week to keep improving. Giving up time with her husband to support his hiking passion was a sacrifice by his wife, but the couple made sure to have enough time together, enough quality time.

The time required for a large volume of physical activity is a challenge for relationships. Less time might mean less contact with friends and loved ones. That could mean less intimacy and closeness and maybe more burden on others who assume responsibility in your absence. People who supported your exercise might start resenting it and see you as self-centered, ungenerous, controlling, or insensitive to the needs of others. If you feel guilty or worried that your family is being neglected, your exercise might start feeling more like stress than joy.

How can you maintain some balance in life so that close relationships and health are both priorities? How can you give back to people who are giving to you? How can you manage stress or guilt about taking care of yourself? ... Quality time.

Quality time is a concept popularized in the 1970s when there was a large increase in dual career families and working parents, especially mothers, worried about the effect of less time at home on their children. The notion was that it is not how much time you spend with your children; it's how you spend that time. Quality over quantity it was said, and born was an idea that helped parents cope with worry and guilt and supposedly would ensure healthy child development.

What is quality time? Generally, it is time spent with family, partners or friends that creates a feeling of closeness by meaningful sharing and connecting emotionally. It's a time when people concentrate on each other without distraction and interruption. If you are busy and even busier now trying to get a lot of exercise hours, quality time will help others to feel good about the relationship and about themselves, and frankly, to be rewarded for putting up with your absence and be willing to keep supporting you. There are two very different strategies for making quality time: quality planned activities and quality moments.

Quality planned activities. Just as you schedule exercise in advance to make sure it happens, plan quality activities with loved ones at times outside of the normal daily routine when you can concentrate on each other. You could plan a special event like a family vacation, weekend ski trip, visit to the aquarium, picnic at the beach, flea market outing, or a romantic getaway. Activities like these can be opportunities for fun, relaxation, and time away from the usual routine. However, it may be difficult to set aside a large block of time often enough.

Ordinary special activities that can be scheduled more frequently would offer more quantity of time as well as quality. Examples are planned activities that can become a weekly tradition such as a family game night, Sunday afternoon television football party, family meeting, religious service, romantic night, or movie night. Find activities that people can look forward to without a long delay. If you think of quality time as a reward to others for patience with your busy schedule, it's more effective to make that reward a short-term consequence. Promising a holiday months into the future is not an effective motivator. Keep in mind also that quality activities imply that you focus your energy on your loved one or friend. Just sitting next to your partner while watching a movie is not necessarily quality time.

Talking about the movie, showing interest in your partner's opinion, cuddling, and not responding to distractions make for a quality experience.

Our family used to call these planned activities, "mandatory fun." That was a playful in-your-face term to our adolescent children who were resistant to doing things as a family. Forcing our kids to spend time with us often worked. But staged recreation isn't always fun. Structured planning adds a burden to an already hectic schedule. It may be hard to find a time block every week or every couple days for quality time. A special outing for the kids or a romantic evening with your partner will not make-up for being gone a lot. But there are many opportunities to interact with loved ones during unplanned, unstructured time. These are quality moments.

Quality moments. Quality moments are times to connect during ordinary daily activities. There are plenty of opportunities in a normal day to take a moment to focus on your friend or family member to ask about their day and share something about yourself. A brief conversation, a moment of togetherness, a little affection go a long way to feel close and show you care. It's the small spontaneous moments like these that occur frequently and are valued in healthy relationships. Quality moments strengthen family and friendship bonds.

Have that heart-to-heart talk with your partner. Catch-up on what is going on in your child's life. Let your friend talk about her work problems. Look for moments when you already are together doing house chores, cooking, working, shopping, helping with homework, saying goodnight. Take advantage of driving time with children when they are a captive audience.

Quality together time does not have to be staged recreation or a special activity. It's anytime you can have a meaningful conversation.

Make it a supportive and nurturing conversation. Be curious about what the person is thinking or doing lately. Listen to the other person; really hear what he or she says. Don't expect to solve their problems, just listen and center on his or her needs or opinions, rather than yours. Share your own thoughts and feelings; reveal something about yourself, but only give advice if asked or it's appropriate.

Make social time, exercise time. Exercise does not have to compete for time with other people. What better way is there to have some fun with friends, family or workmates than to enjoy a good outdoor activity or workout together away from distractions of the daily routine? Sports and physical recreation can trigger intense emotional experiences, especially if doing something novel, adventurous or challenging. Emotions like thrill, excitement, fatigue, pain, and feelings of accomplishment. Sharing these with other people creates a sense of closeness. Exercise is a stress reliever. It decreases tension and consequently can be a good time to connect with people, to have an intimate and more relaxed conversation. Exercise time with people is quality time. The benefits are good for relationships and importantly, for your desire to keep exercising.

Social exercise. Social exercise is social support. Schedule exercise with other people especially when you are having trouble making yourself go alone. An appointment with a friend to exercise is a commitment that will make you want to follow through.

Personally, I enjoy a nice long hike or ride all by myself. It's a good time to think and take care of business while moving. But most days I'm really glad I have some exercise buddies. Were it not for our scheduled group rides, I might not ride as much as I want to. A few of my cycling friends only ride when they can hook-up with other people. They need other people to be motivated. No wonder that we have a tradition of saying "Thank you" at the end of a ride, as we peel off one-by-one in the direction of our homes. We depend on each other to exercise.

Dogs can be good social supports because they need regular exercise too. Use the dog as an exercise companion and excuse for a good walk. Don't just stand there and throw the ball. Walk with the dog and increase the length of time or frequency that you dog walk. Your dog certainly won't mind. It turns out that people usually walk faster and further with dogs than with human companions or when walking alone.

If your friends are not available to join you in person, they still can exercise with you virtually. Create a social network with a social media or fitness app that allows you to send notifications or post your diary and allows friends to post comments back to you.

Let exercise friends push you outside your comfort zone. Use peer pressure to your advantage. It's harder to say no and easier to take more risks around other people. Exercise with someone or a group that will push you to work harder or try something you might not on your own. A team of friends who commits to do an event like a team triathlon can make you go beyond your usual physical limitation. People who cycle, ski, or run together, no matter how good friends they are, can be very competitive at the moment. In my group rides every little hill or city limit sign becomes a competition zone. It's a fun, friendly way to practice high intensity exercise intervals.

Some of my women clients started walking or hiking with their husbands, not just for quality time, but to force themselves to pick-up their pace and to develop some speed. In contrast, I have athletic friends who actually need an easy day of exercise to recover from hard training. They make themselves take it easy by saving that time for a ride or walk with their spouses who exercise at a calmer level. I've worked with many clients who wanted to try something new like weight training or swimming in a fitness center, but they were intimidated until a friend volunteered to be their exercise buddy and show them how.

You don't need live friends to inspire you with an exercise challenge. There are social media apps for walking, running, and cycling that can monitor your route, distance, elevation gain, and time via GPS or manual data input. That information is posted to an online fitness community where you can compare yourself to friends who use the app or other locals or even pro athletes who do the same route. An anonymous forum can make competition against other exercisers feel less risky and stressful. Networks that create challenges like to go a certain distance or climb a certain number of feet hiking can attract thousands of people around the world. Seeing your result on the board and receiving praise for your achievement from other users can be a great motivator. Without fail, there will be others who are more fit and ambitious than you. Use helpful self-talk when you compare yourself.

Combine exercise with social events. What is the custom for outings and get-togethers with your family and friends? Do you ever plan physically active times? Is it normal for people around you to share sports and physical recreation? Are your dates outdoorsy and active? Do you have any traditions at work that involve a physical outing? Do you and your partner de-compress with an evening walk? Or do you spend too much time with the family shopping and cruising the stores on the weekends? Are visits with your friends always for lunch and drinks? Are camping trips with other families spent sitting around the picnic table? Are holiday celebrations all about food and lazing about?

Turn family events, visits with friends and workdays into

exercise opportunities. Compared to a discussion sitting down, people disclose more and enjoy personal talks more while being physically active together. If you are into walking, invite your partner to join you. If you are trying to hike more, create some outings with the entire family for a nature experience. Train the kids to expect something outdoorsy as a family before sedentary activities happen. Instead of hanging out in the staff room at lunch, have the conversation while moving or at the company fitness center. On holidays, organize a nice walk or backyard game before the big meal. For an active evening out with your partner or friends, try dancing. How about playing a real football game with friends instead of fantasy football on the computer. Think about converting sedentary social pastimes of luncheons, dinners, and TV sports watching to something more active. If your children are very young, put them in the stroller or backpack and take a long hike or walk.

Reflections On Social Support

Exercise is a time occupying activity and consequently will eventually affect people around you. Some negotiation with potential social support persons might be necessary to get them on your side. You know what you need to do for a healthy lifestyle; don't sacrifice yourself. Find ways to include others in your physical activity. Physical recreation elicits emotions and when shared with other people it can create a sense of mutual closeness.

Chapter 10:
Vary Your Exercise Intensity

Your assignment in this chapter is to develop an exercise routine with different levels of intensity. Intensity refers to how much work is being done during exercise and how hard the exercise feels to you. The amount of oxygen and fuel you use, the calories you burn, your heart rate, and the muscle strength you need are influenced by intensity. Repetition of the same exercise is good at the beginning for the sake of forming a habit and also to adapt physically to being more active. However, what happens if you always do the same thing and never vary your routine?

Advantages And Disadvantages Of Routine Exercise

Most people who are trying to get back into an exercise habit start with some regular routine. I've worked with many clients who gradually built up to a nice 30-minute walk around their neighborhood five days a week. Many of my clients would get back to the fitness center and do a cardio and weight training workout three or four days a week. Without awareness of why, people are attracted to repeating the same workout day after day because it helps to make that exercise easier and more familiar – closer to being automatic. Repetition and practice is the key to learning.

Repeating one type of exercise intensity helps your body learn and adapt to that particular type of physical work. This happens because physical performance consists of behavioral and physiological responses that are subject to a learning process like any response. When you walk at a certain speed along a certain terrain, you learn how to move and balance yourself, how quickly to step in order to maintain your usual pace, how to adjust your footing as the walking surface changes. These responses become automatic with practice. At the same time, physiological processes out of your awareness are also learning to adapt to the work demand; processes such as muscle strength, absorption of oxygen, and the utilization of nutrients to sustain your physical work. With practice, your body becomes more efficient, more capable and you feel less tired. It learned how to do that walk.

One disadvantage of doing that same old walk over and over is that your body will only know that one thing. It won't be prepared for demands to function in a different way. That's a consequence of practicing just one type of workout. Let's say you enjoy that nightly walk on flat streets, walking one and one-half miles in 30 minutes. You're an expert in that walk. But what might happen when you are away from home and walk a hilly neighborhood with steep streets? You'll feel really tired. Or what if you spend a vacation in Washington D.C. and want to visit the museums and monuments around the National Mall? That could take a full day of walking. You might not be able to walk that much or if you do, you'd feel really tired. If you never vary your routine, you'll have trouble adapting to different physical and psychological demands.

Why Vary Your Exercise Intensity?

The beginning steps to make yourself exercise are to increase the frequency and total time being physically active. The quality of exercise is not important from a behavioral point of view, because the purpose of a gradual increase is to strengthen your commitment and begin a habit. If you have reached that magic number of four days a week, you are ready to start refining the quality of your activity and bring your fitness to a higher level.

I am going to recommend that you create a weekly schedule of exercise at different intensities that includes long sessions of activity that promote endurance, shorter sessions that teach you speed and strength, and other sessions to help recover or just have fun. These different workouts should be phased in gradually, depending where you are at the present time, using an aerobic type of exercise. Later I will also recommend that you create more variety in the type of exercise that you do (see Chapter 12, Vary Your Type of Exercise). You can check that chapter for ideas on which activities are appropriate for the aerobic intensity training about to be presented here. Variety creates better fitness, but the emphasis in this book is on creating a strong habit. Variety makes your exercise habit stronger.

Be prepared for different physical demands. An advantage of varying exercise intensity is, you learn different types of physical work and consequently, you are prepared for different physical demands. I say learn because the performance of an exercise and adaptation are learned behavior, physiological and behavioral responses, that come with practice. You have to go faster if you want to go faster. You have to go longer if you want to go longer. With practice, you can enjoy different degrees of intensity without feeling excessively tired or risking injury. Being capable of different intensities makes you adaptable so you can exercise as hard or easy as needed in the situation. The more situations you can handle, the more outside of your normal exercise environment, the stronger your exercise habit will be. The strength of a behavior depends on the number of situations in which it is practiced.

Here are some examples of training at different intensities and adapting to circumstances.

You went to Washington, D.C. and walked six hours. Although that was a new record for your longest walk, you weren't that tired because you had been doing a three-hour endurance hike once a week at home.

You normally walk a mile in 20 minutes, but you wanted to join a walking group that is faster. You started doing speed intervals a couple times a week to practice a faster pace of 15-minute miles. After feeling more comfortable with 15 minutes, you went on the group walk. It was a challenge but you were able to keep up reasonably well.

You went to San Francisco for vacation. Good thing you had been doing some walking intervals on steep hills at your county park. Walking San Francisco was like a full day of strength training.

You were so enthused about exercising again, that instead of beginning with walking, you started running five days a week. A friend convinced you to not overdo it and to have one easy recovery exercise day a week, especially to not run. You added a slow walking day. That helped you enjoy visiting your elderly aunt whose idea of exercise was a stroll through her neighborhood.

Add purpose and interest to exercise. When you follow a training plan to exercise at different intensities, every day is different. Instead of five of the same old walks each week, you will have to figure out how to get a good long endurance walk as well as the two harder days and some fun outings. Instead of one big goal, five walks, you have five different goals. Every day has a specific physical and psychological benefit. That adds interest and a sense of purpose to the week.

There's a feeling of accomplishment as you tick off the different types of workouts, one by one. You might have some hard days every week, but you can look forward to relief, because there are easy, fun days too. You will have earned those days when you stick to your schedule. That sequence of hard days, followed by easy days increases the likelihood you'll do the hard days in the first instance.

Here are some examples of not getting bored or stale with exercise because you have variety.

You did your speed, strength, and endurance days all in a row. Now you feel relieved that the hard work is behind you for the week and you look forward to going easy the next couple days.
You woke up today thinking, what kind of day will this be today? What is left to accomplish this week? You kind of enjoy the choices you have.
A friend calls you to do a long hike. Perfect. You were thinking of doing an easy day, but hiking with your friend will be a good motivation for an endurance workout. Taking it easy the next day will be your reward.
It's the day for the group walk. You need a recovery day, so instead of walking with the faster walkers, you hang toward the back and take it easy. That gives you a chance to talk with a different group of people.
Today is your day to do some intervals on the elliptical machine. It's so much more interesting and challenging to alternate medium and intense periods than to keep up a steady pace like most other days.

Be flexible. It's good to be creative and flexible. The more you have to tailor exercise episodes to circumstances, the more able you will be to keep exercising when you are out of your normal environment.

The more you can be flexible, the better you will be able to revise your exercise plans when unexpected interferences would otherwise make you think of skipping exercise. Although it's not ideal to improvise, sometimes you must. And having a variety of types of workouts in your repertoire gives you a way to find something that fits the situation. Check these examples.

You were supposed to swim for 60 minutes today, but you had a schedule change and there's not enough time. To save time, you decided to do some sprint intervals and finish in 30 minutes.
It's a travel day, so you don't have the bike for your usual long ride. No problem, you used the day as a recovery day and did an easy walk in-between business meetings.
You still had to get your endurance day for the week, but the family wanted to do a hike – less time than you needed. So you ran to the trailhead to meet your wife and children and then hiked, giving you the total time you needed.
You planned to do some high intensity intervals on the elliptical machine. After a couple attempts at a higher resistance, you realize you're too tired from yesterday's endurance workout, so you decided to try intervals tomorrow and spend today at a medium steady effort to help recover.

Improve your fitness. Physical fitness is not just the absence of disease, but a state of health and well-being; the ability to function effectively and without undue fatigue in daily work, leisure activities and emergency situations. Increases in fitness eventually will lessen if you repeat the same exercise over and over. You need to vary the routine if you want to keep improving. Having some days with higher intensity exercise makes you faster and stronger. Longer episodes of exercise will increase endurance. The purpose of high intensity and endurance days is to increase the body's physical work beyond what it is used to. The purpose of easier, recovery days is to reduce the risk of injury and psychological burnout. Alternating stressing the body and recovering forces the body to adapt by developing more efficient and capable physical responses.

Here are some of the important physical improvements you can expect with a well-organized training plan. Each of these changes makes exercise feel less of an effort and thereby acts as a reward for following the plan. And since it does not take long to feel more physically fit, the reward is short term. The best motivator for exercise is built-in short-term rewards.

Heart and lung function. Your heart muscle will become stronger which increases the amount of blood it can pump while doing so at a lower heart rate. The blood will have more red blood cells and flow with less resistance, so much more oxygen and nutrients will be transported to muscles. The muscles of the respiratory system also become stronger, increasing the amount of oxygen to fuel your activity. As a result, exercise will take less effort, will feel more comfortable and you will become faster and be able to go longer before stopping. More waste products from exercise in the muscles will be carried away, which will make you feel less sore. Cholesterol levels become more healthy.

Muscles. The size of the muscles used for your exercise increase. That makes you stronger and faster. As your body composition changes by increasing muscle tissue, your metabolic rate increases. That means you'll burn more calories even when not exercising because muscle requires more energy than fat tissue. Muscles become better able to extract and use oxygen from blood to burn as fuel. Small blood vessels and special cells in muscle fibers increase in number, supplying more nutrients. The byproducts of strenuous muscle contractions are removed more efficiently. As a result, you feel more energetic, less tired, and less sore. Musculoskeletal problems involving pain or disability are improved.

Thermoregulation. Thermoregulation is the ability to keep body temperature within certain boundaries. Many people hate to sweat when exercising, but sweating is an adaptive response to control body heat. The problem underlying discomfort in the unfit exerciser is too much body heat. As fitness improves you actually sweat more, because the sweat glands react sooner to the onset of exercise. In addition, more blood flows to the small blood vessels supplying the skin, which helps to shed heat. Therefore, you become more efficient at controlling body heat and the unpleasant experience of being overheated is eliminated.

Metabolic rate. Exercise burns calories. But most calories are burned to maintain normal bodily processes in a neutral or resting state, the resting metabolic rate. As you develop more lean muscle tissue, your metabolism will increase. The lower metabolic rate of older adults is attributable to declining muscle mass. Starting to exercise again can reverse this process. Strenuous exercise intervals burn more calories than moving at a constant speed and they stimulate an increase in resting metabolic rate beyond that caused by changes in muscle mass. These metabolic increases result in weight loss and decreases in abdominal size.

Nutrition. Exercise requires energy from nutrients. As you exercise, your body will start using internally stored energy beginning with carbohydrate, most of which is accumulated in muscle. Muscles become better able to store carbohydrate as your fitness improves, but the supply is limited. If you exercise continuously for a long session, stored carbohydrate will diminish. Then the body begins to switch to body fat stores to make energy. Again, becoming physically fit improves the ability to break down and release this energy. With more fuel efficiency, you go longer, feel less tired, and are less likely to have unpleasant mental symptoms.

Mental function. Feedback from body movements and physical effort creates growth in the neural pathways from the body to the brain. Reaction times, sensory awareness of the body in space and movement, and adjustments in movement in order to maintain balance and prevent falls all improve.

Blood flow and nutrients to the brain increase with more physical activity. Brain size, neural connections, and brain activity increase and brain deterioration decreases in conjunction with more exercise. Psychologically, performance on cognitive and memory testing is improved, positive emotions increase, negative emotions decrease, and reactions to stress lessen. These changes do not necessarily make exercise physically easier, but they could give the extra mental energy and capacity to cope with exercise when it's added to an already busy schedule.

Measure Your Exercise Intensity

To know if you are varying your exercise intensity, you need a way to measure it. Without measuring, you are just estimating. When it comes to health and fitness, people tend to distort estimates in their favor; usually in the direction of thinking a workout was more intense than it really was. Measurement of intensity gives you more accurate feedback about your exercise and like any form of self-monitoring, it triggers behavior change in the desired direction. In this case, knowing your heart rate will encourage you to reach the intensity that is right for your fitness goals and level of fitness.

The most practical and convenient measure of exercise intensity is your pulse or heart rate in the form of beats per minute. This simple physical measure is the closest estimate of other physical responses to exercise that would require being tested in a sports medicine laboratory.

Calculate your heart rate zones. Exercise intensity can be broken into five zones of heart rate. The boundary of each zone is a percent of your maximum heart rate. Maximum heart rate during exercise can be determined in a sports medicine or fitness laboratory on a treadmill or other indoor exercise machine. A stress test for heart disease uses a similar test procedure, but normally does not continue to the point of discovering how rapid your heart can beat before exhaustion. The alternative and most practical way to determine your maximum heart rate is to estimate it with a simple formula.

Step one: estimate your maximum heart rate. Your estimated maximum heart rate is 220 minus your age = _____.

Step two: calculate the lower and upper limits of each heart rate zone. Multiply your estimated maximum heart rate by the percentages of maximum for the range or lower and upper limits of each zone. For example, if you are 50 years old, your estimated maximum is 170 beats per minutes. The lower limit of Zone 1 would be 170 X .50 (50% of maximum) = 85 beats per minute. Write the results in Figure 10.1. Next, compute 170 X .59 and write the answer 100 for the upper limit of Zone 1. There are other formulas to estimate maximum heart rate and cutoffs for heart rate zones. None is a perfect estimate compared to laboratory testing and all define exercise zones somewhat arbitrarily.

Zone	Percent of maximum heart rate	My heart rate range (lower & upper limits)	
Z1	50% to 59%	_____ to	_____
Z2	60% to 69%	_____ to	_____
Z3	70% to 79%	_____ to	_____
Z4	80% to 89%	_____ to	_____
Z5	90% to 100%	_____ to	_____

Figure 10.1 Calculate the boundaries of your heart rate zones as a function of estimated maximum heart rate.

How to measure heart rate. An objective, accurate measure of heart rate is with a heart rate monitor, normally a heart rate sensor strap worn around the chest that transmits wirelessly either to a special wristwatch computer, a bicycle computer or to a smartphone app. Some activity trackers worn on the wrist can estimate heart rate. Most indoor exercise machines have a handgrip that can detect pulse and display it on the machine information window. Stopping exercise to measure your pulse is not as accurate as the instantaneous feedback from a heart rate monitor. By the time you find and count your pulse, your heart rate will have dropped.

The most basic information from these devices is live moment-to-moment heart rate. Other capabilities that can be helpful are an audio alert when you have reached a heart rate zone you want to target and an analysis of your exercise episode by reporting the time you spent in each heart rate zone. Just knowing your heart beats per minute as you exercise is enough at the beginning.

If you do not have a heart rate monitor or you are on medication for a heart condition that slows your heart rate such as beta-blockers or calcium channel blockers, you should try this alternative scale of exercise intensity, a simple scale of breathing intensity (Figure 10.2). As you are exercising, talk out loud long enough to see how increased breathing might affect your speaking. There is a pretty good correlation between these symptoms of breathing intensity and levels of heart rate.

Zone	Breathing
Z1	Able to speak without trouble.
Z2	Can speak, but takes some effort.
Z3	Hard to speak in complete sentences without taking a breath.
Z4	Breathing too rapidly to say more than a couple of words.
Z5	Can't speak at all. Breathing fast and hard with snot and drool

Figure 10.2 A scale of breathing intensity to estimate heart rate zone.

Notice the other symptoms of Zone 5 – snot and drool. These telltale signs of near maximum effort happen because intense exercise produces more mucous in the nose and mouth. Additionally, people tend to open their mouths to facilitate rapid breathing, which encourages drooling. Not a very appealing picture, but to those sports participants who like to push themselves, snot and drool are a badge of honor.

A new exercise diary. The best start and motivation for varying exercise intensity is to keep a record. So, in addition to the amount of exercise time in your diary, start recording the intensity of each exercise episode. The new diary (Figure 10.4) simply adds one column in which you can write something about intensity. At a minimum, write the heart rate zone or zones in which you spent the most time. You do need to write other heart rate zones that were unrelated to the purpose of the workout, for instance, Zone 1 while warming up. Momentarily slips into higher zones also do not need to be recorded. For the high intensity days, write something to keep track of your progress on doing intervals, such as the heart rate zone, time and number of intervals, and type of interval. See Figure 10.3 for examples. It might seem like a lot of trouble to record extra detail, but written information on your behavior gives you extra power to change.

week starting June 1	exercise	time	intensity
Monday	walk the dog	16 min	Z1
Tuesday	walk to market	24 min	Z2
Wednesday	Hike the state park	75 min	Z2-3, two 5 min Z4 intervals climbing
Thursday	Bicycle ride	28 min	Z2, couple short speed intervals Zone 3

Figure 10.3 A daily record of exercise should include the intensity & type of intervals if applicable

week starting	exercise (if more than one bout of exercise, list separately)	time	intensity
Monday			
Tuesday			
Wednesday			
Thursday			
Friday			
Saturday			
Sunday			

number of days with exercise _____   total time _____

Figure 10.4 Record heart rate zone for feedback on your intensity

Know Your Heart Rate Zones

Each heart rate zone does something special for your fitness and enjoyment; each feels different. Getting to know the differences between exercise zones will encourage you to use and enjoy them and to take more control of your exercise. If you know what to expect, if you recognize the normal feelings and sensations of high intensity levels, you might feel more at ease and less worried about working hard.

Zone 1. This level is easy, but still is an exercise intensity that will increase fitness. The increased blood flow and easy movement reduces stiffness and improves function of the joints. Good for the beginner, Zone 1 is a way to move and improve overall health without feeling overly tired. When exercising with other people at this intensity you can feel comfortable – it's good for socializing at the same time you are accomplishing something for your health. Zone 1 also is used for warming up and cooling down during a more intense exercise session. Active recovery or rest days should be spent mainly in Zone 1.

Zone 2. This zone is the lower end of the aerobic range, the intensity at which exercise increases the need for oxygen and begins to improve heart and lung function. Most aerobic type exercise is spent in Zone 2, whether you are a regular exerciser or you are beginning to increase. Although this intensity demands more physically than Zone 1, it still will feel easy for most people, easy enough that it is a good level for endurance or long, slow workouts. You can still speak fluently in Zone 2, so it's a fine way to socialize while exercising. As fitness improves, you should be able to work in this zone for hours. Zone 2 is good for losing weight not only because people are capable of staying at this intensity for a long while, but because much of its fuel comes from stored body fat.

Zone 3. Increasing to Zone 3 puts you in the moderately

intense range, which is the one most commonly targeted in aerobic exercise. Best for overall fitness, Zone 3 stimulates more cardio-respiratory capacity and boosts muscular strength as well. To work in this zone requires moving at a faster, harder pace, but with experience it's an effort that you should be able to continue for a long while without feeling pain or soreness. Zone 3 will help with weight control once you can go longer at this intensity, because the body will emphasize stored fat for energy. It's harder to have a fluent conversation at this level. On exercise machines in the fitness center, you should not be able to read or concentrate on television at this intensity.

Zone 4. Exercising in Zone 4 feels hard and tiring and cannot be sustained for a long while like the lower heart rate zones. The heavy breathing can be intimidating. But what usually makes people pull out of Zone 4 is the feeling of muscle fatigue and inability to keep going at this level. In Zones 1 to 3, the regular exerciser could go indefinitely and usually stops because time is up. After a while the feeling in Zone 4 is "this is too hard" to go any longer. The benefit of working this hard is you learn how to put out an intense effort for short periods of time. Your muscles adapt to strenuous effort. They become stronger, more powerful and better able to eliminate the physical causes of fatigue. Working in this zone is beneficial occasionally for most regular exercisers and especially for people who want to improve their performance for competition or recreational athletic events. If you want to go fast or climb hills at a good pace, you need practice with Zone 4.

Zone 5. This zone is for very short, hard efforts, a sprint or moving as fast as you can. Unlike being in the lower zones, here you know you cannot work any harder. And you cannot keep it up for more than a few seconds or minutes. Your muscles can feel like they are on fire and you are panting as fast as you can. Zone 5 is the anaerobic range, a point at which a byproduct of intense muscular action builds up in the bloodstream and creates a feeling of fatigue. Working in this zone may not be necessary for health, but it helps people develop power, muscle speed. This is important for intense bursts of effort at crucial moments such as in athletic competition or emergency situations. Simply working in Zone 5 gives you a feeling of vitality and having guts.

There are two ways to look at exercise intensity. One is the type of activity – how fast, how steep, how much resistance. The other is the body's response to the activity. The person who has not been exercising much might feel out of breath when walking quickly. Whereas the more experienced fit exerciser might need to run before breathing hard. The activities are different, but the physical efforts by the exercisers are the same. Over time, the new exerciser will be able to move faster without having to increase the physical effort. Because the intensity of activity is relative – what is fast to one person is slow to another – the more important measure of intensity is something like heart rate. Knowing your heart rate or heart rate zone allows you to compare one activity to another and to adjust the intensity of activity as your fitness improves.

Basic Concepts In Varying Exercise Intensity

Create a weekly schedule. The objective is to develop a routine of working out at different levels of intensity each week. Figure 10.5 shows a breakdown of exercise time and intensity for a walker who is up to a desirable amount of exercise, about six hours and seven days per week.

You should have two "hard" days that include high intensity intervals of strenuous work. These are shorter exercise episodes designed to practice speed (e.g., walking a fast pace on level terrain) or strength (walking hills). Hard days are usually separated by at least one normal or easier exercise day to aid recovery. The example shows hard days on Tuesday and Thursday with a fun, medium day in-between and a shorter, fun day before the endurance day. Fun, light to medium intensity days should be your normal type of exercise, focusing mainly on putting in the time and having fun. An endurance episode is at a moderate, rather than strenuous intensity, and two or more times longer than your usual exercise. This example shows an endurance walk to be twice as long as the next longest episodes of the week (120 minutes vs. 60 minutes). The recovery day usually comes after you have done your hard work for the week, at the end of the week or the very beginning of the following week. Recovery is your usual exercise at a much lower, leisurely intensity.

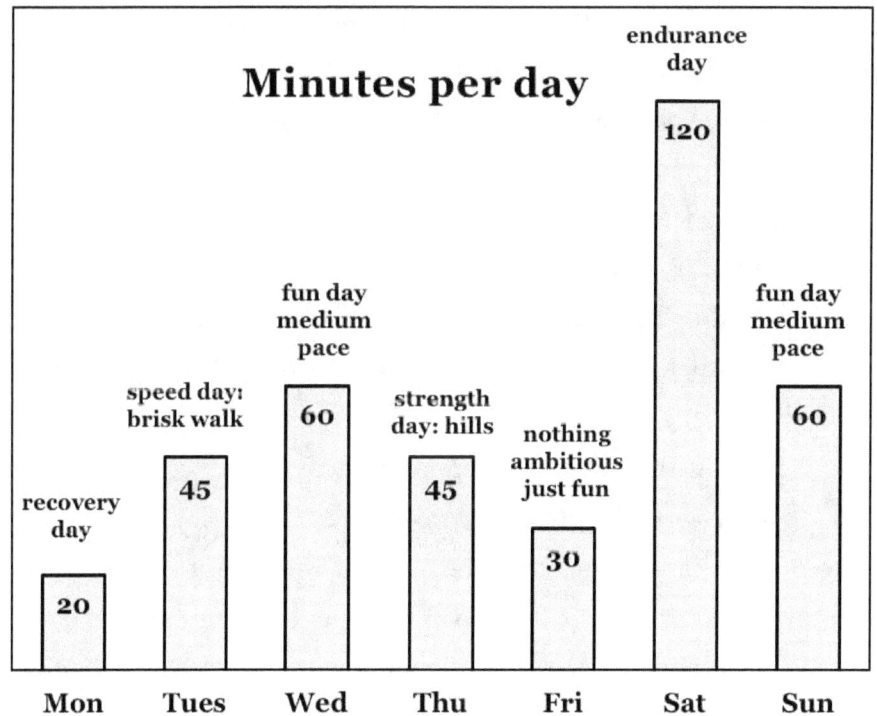

Figure 10.5. Example of a varied walking routine for total of 6 hrs. 20 min. per week. Make every exercise day different to increase your fitness.

Adjust the schedule according to the number of days you are regularly exercising at the present time. (See below for suggestions.) If you are weight training or practicing yoga or other exercise that is not aerobic, you can mix them into a schedule of varied exercise intensity. Try counting them as medium, fun days or even a recovery day. For good overall fitness, you will need at least several days of an aerobic type activity in addition to any other type that you enjoy.

Endurance day. When you are regularly exercising on four days a week, the next best step is to have one day a week with a long exercise session. Most people have plenty of short days, rest days, or medium hard days, but generally they are missing an endurance day. Adding one endurance day a week will boost your fitness and trigger several changes that will help make exercise a strong habit. One long exercise session per week is a great way to build your total exercise time toward that important goal of six hours. Adding high intensity intervals is important too, but endurance training is easier and more natural and consequently it is a good way to start varying exercise intensity. After you have had some success with endurance training, you should be ready to move ahead with high intensity work. Do not expect to establish a schedule like Figure 10.5 all at once. Gradually phase-in the variety. Begin with increasing your endurance.

Duration of endurance episodes. Our biological ancestors evolved to be capable of extensive physical work, so it should not be unnatural or unusually stressful to move around and use muscle power for hours at a time. However, labor saving devices, mechanized transportation and sedentary occupations have eliminated the need for long doses of activity. Most people squeeze in a little exercise around work and other daily responsibilities, because there is no natural requirement to do more. How can you create a long block of time and make yourself keep going without stopping? Here are some tips to build endurance.

A reasonable goal at the beginning is lengthen one exercise day to twice as long as normal. People who are ready for this typically have been exercising 20 to 40 minutes at a time. Perhaps you can handle doubling that time right now. Otherwise, gradually add time, five, ten, or fifteen minutes to one of your usual bouts of exercise until you have created a nice, long endurance day. Use your watch to measure the increases. Don't guess, otherwise you risk not adding real increases. If there are logistic problems to longer stretches of exercise or you find it difficult physically, make the increases very gradual. But keep increasing. If you only have one form of exercise, such as walking, it is especially important to increase slowly in order to avoid injury. Your exercise record is a way to keep track of your longest episode of exercise, a personal record of sorts. Build on that. Keep setting a new record for longest walk, longest hike, longest swim, etc.

The limit to continuous physical activity is very high. So, after doubling your normal exercise time, increasing to a half-day or full day of activity is not an unreasonable goal. This kind of endurance will boost your fitness even more and deepen your habit. Hopefully with practice, you'll discover that physically you can handle it and that you can re-orient your lifestyle to make it happen. I find it can require months for some people to move from a "short" endurance episode of an hour and a half to a full day. Be persistent. Add time. Find ways to make a day a physically active day.

As you gradually increase the length of your endurance day, you might start feeling bored doing the same thing continuously. Indoor workouts on fitness machines are especially difficult to tolerate for long. Personally, even with heavy video distraction, I was never able to ride an indoor bicycle trainer for more than an hour during the Vermont winters. Instead of making your workout even more tiring mentally than it will be physically, try combining a couple activities, one after another to make your endurance time. Using different parts of your body with two activities is a good way to reduce the risk of injury. Doing two separate bouts of exercise hours apart on a single day is not an endurance workout. Endurance training is long, continuous exercise. If you combine different types, combine them without a significant break. Some examples from my clients are:

Walk to and from the fitness center to do your usual workout.
Do your indoor video exercise and then go outside for your usual walking loop
Meet your family at the park by riding your bike there and then join them for the Frisbee game and picnic.
Instead of alternating days of yoga and weight training, pick one day when you do both, one after the other

There are many ways to devote a full day to exercise. I found that almost everyone in my weight control program was able to walk all day on vacation. The challenge is how to create a full exercise day on a routine basis. That requires some extra re-organization of your schedule as well as some courage to try something more ambitious than normal. Some examples of activities that can keep you busy all day are: golf game, day hike, century bike ride, skiing, ball game, stream fishing, or sightseeing walk.

Earlier when talking about self-monitoring (Chapter 3), I recommended not counting chores of daily life in your exercise diary.

Although vigorous housework and home projects can have the same calorie burn or fitness effect as formal exercise, I want you to measure exercise because that is the harder behavior to increase and the one needed to develop a truly active lifestyle. Nonetheless, if you are struggling to find something you can do half or all day, at the beginning it would be okay to use a house project for your endurance workout so long as you spend a good portion of time in the aerobic zone. Gardening and yard work are the second most popular leisure time activities, behind walking. Plan a long day of gardening and move quickly and vigorously so you approximate the effort you would make on a long walk or hike. Make this a temporary substitute while you develop an endurance form of exercise.

Intensity of endurance episodes. Most of your endurance workout should be in the aerobic range, mainly in Zone 2. Some work in Zone 3 is okay. Try to avoid pushing yourself into Zone 4 and certainly not into Zone 5. The point of an endurance day is to practice long times of reasonably low level of physical activity. You should feel spent after your workout, but not stressed or sore like you might after high intensity intervals.

Since an endurance session is long, there is no need to hurry to get your heart rate into the aerobic range. Take your time to warm up. After reaching Zone 2, stay there, but let yourself reach into Zone 3 as necessitated by circumstances. For example, if you're doing a day hike and have some hills, it's likely your heart rate will increase beyond Zone 2. Don't let it go too high. You might have to slow your walking pace, for instance, to keep your heart rate down.

As your exercise time increases and you reach one hour, two hours or more of continuous work, you must remain hydrated. Drink before exercise and after. If you will be on the move for a couple hours or longer, take liquid and a quick energy snack with you.

Coping with endurance exercise. Long continuous exercise at a low intensity prepares you for other types of long physical activity, such as walking on vacation or a full day of yard work. You learn physical endurance. You also learn mental endurance, because psychologically you must sustain interest and persistence with exercise for a long while.

Two common issues people struggle with are feeling bored as time goes on and thinking about other things to do instead of exercising. Either one of these pop into consciousness via self-talk. If you start telling yourself "This is boring. I'm getting tired of this. I can't wait until the 3 hours are over," your persistence is at risk. If you start thinking about taking time away from something else, you might not reach the time goal for an endurance day. You have the power to revise how you talk to yourself about boredom or time conflicts to make it more possible to finish your endurance workout. Reread the chapter on self-talk to prepare yourself for exercise friendly answers.

To deal with boredom or low motivation, design endurance days to be interesting or create an incentive to complete the workout. It's easy to get on a treadmill for 20 minutes, but to keep walking for an hour you need a good immediate payoff, not a distant hope for better fitness. Try designing an outing to reach a meaningful destination: walk a good distance to the restaurant; instead of driving to shop, walk and carry your purchases in a backpack; use your bicycle instead of the car to visit relatives. A classic incentive or reward for hiking is to reach the summit of a hill or other viewpoint. It is a draw to keep going. The feeling of accomplishment to reach a landmark is more powerful than ticking off laps around the neighborhood. Plus the return trip downhill or back to the car usually goes faster or at least feels faster because the end is in sight. Organize some fun leisure time activity that will double as your endurance episode. A day of field games with the children gives your exercise time and serves an important purpose. Schedule your endurance workout with other people so you have some social pressure and social distraction to keep going. Group rides, walks, and hikes are popular for the motivation and social effects. By necessity, long endurance exercise teaches one to overcome boredom.

A classic way to get into endurance training is sign-up for a fund-raising event such as a diabetes or MS ride or walk. Usually one must prepare for the long event by building up endurance during the weeks or months leading to the big day. Making a commitment by paying a registration or raising donations from other people makes it more likely you'll follow through.

Endurance is time occupying and you must learn to deal with time conflicts and replace other activities with exercise. You can't do a long hike every Saturday and still spend the day shopping, watching ballgames, reading or taking a nap. Those behaviors will have to be re-scheduled or eliminated. With endurance added to your routine, exercise is not just an hour here or there, it's a lifestyle that requires letting go of activities that don't contribute to your fitness and physical recreation. You have to make some choices. An endurance day is the best way to start that process.

High intensity days. Advanced exercisers who are past the habit formation stage are more likely to have high intensity days. Is this because being advanced prepares you to exercise harder or because high intensity exercise creates a stronger habit? I think it's both. After accumulating some experience with regular exercise, physically and mentally you should be capable of trying something more difficult. At the same time, the fitness boost and mental toughness from intense exercise will make you want to exercise more.

High intensity workouts alternate between intervals of strenuous work and recovery. Adding high intensity to your routine is appropriate if you have been able to exercise above your aerobic threshold, in Zone 2 or higher, and you have already or are developing an endurance day. If for instance, you are exercising on four days, you should have one endurance and one high intensity day. If you exercise daily or almost every day, you are ready to do a high intensity workout twice a week.

Begin with a warm up period approximately one-quarter to one-half the duration of the activity. Continue your exercise long enough to feel energetic. Not giving yourself enough time to warm up will prevent your body from reaching the intensity needed for a good fitness benefit. These are shorter exercise days, but be careful to not make them so short that you are not prepared to work hard. Warm up should begin below the aerobic threshold and move into Zone 2 and 3 aerobic ranges before you start your intervals of high intensity.

High intensity intervals are short periods of intense exercise that should push your body beyond your comfort zone. Intervals train your body to function at an intense level by taking it in small doses; small doses of vigorous muscle action and speed, which in time lead to going faster or harder for longer periods. There is no single definition of an interval. You can design intervals to target different abilities and you can vary the intensity, duration, number of repetitions, and the recovery in-between intervals. The variety of possibilities allows you to adjust interval training to keep advancing your fitness and to make these workouts interesting.

Type of interval. To make it simple at this time, think of workouts that emphasize strength or speed during aerobic exercise. A strength workout for a walker, runner, hiker, cyclist, in-line skater, cross country skier or anyone doing exercise primarily using leg power outdoors would be climbing hills or rises in the landscape. If you live in flat terrain, exercising into a stiff headwind is a strength workout. If you are an indoor exerciser, you would use more strength by increasing the resistance or incline on the machine to simulate a hill. Swimmers can do laps with just arm pulls or a kickboard. Rowers can increase pressure on the oars or extend the knees forcefully on a sliding seat. Leg and arm speeds are normally lower during strength intervals, because the resistance to movement is great.

Speed intervals increase the speed of leg and arm movement by picking up the pace, usually on level or gently rolling terrain. Increase the speed by moving faster, at a brisk pace. Heading downwind on a windy day allows higher leg and arm speed. For indoor workouts, reduce the resistance or incline of the machine and move faster or set the treadmill speed to a higher level. Rowers can increase the rate of strokes.

Duration of intervals. The length of an interval is a function of the intensity of work. The greater the intensity, the shorter the interval. At the beginning, you should practice moderate increases in effort that you can sustain for a couple minutes before having to rest. Later, as your fitness improves and you have the mental strength to cope with intense effort, you could practice intervals as short as five seconds near maximum effort or long intervals in the high aerobic range.

This table (Figure 10.6) shows a sample of schedules for intervals to give you an idea of the timing. Easier or moderately intense intervals are listed first. Use a watch and follow the time specifications exactly. For example, build up speed or the steepness of a climb until you approach the higher intensity; check the time. Continue until you reach the end of the interval and then slow down to an easy pace for the exact time allowed for recovery. Repeat the high intensity, recover, and repeat as often as specified. A set consists of several repetitions with a recovery or medium interlude. At first, do just one set of intervals, followed by recovery and medium effort and then cool down.

Notice that the total time of intense intervals in these examples is very short. The sample "hard" days in Figure 10.5 are 45 minutes, but you might only spend 12 minutes total in a high heart rate zone. These short bouts of vigorous exercise improve health a lot. Long bouts over ten minutes of high intensity are healthy too, of course. And they are useful if your recreation outings are long and hard. Long mountainous hikes, long climbs on a bicycle, endurance runs etc., can put you in Zone 4 for an hour at a time. Practicing long intervals prepares you to perform in those situations. But you still will improve health with far shorter intense intervals.

If you are new to interval training, a gradual and systematic increase in the workload will help you cope with the extra effort and will result in physical improvement without risk of injury or feeling too tired and burned-out. Allow several weeks of one set of intervals before you add a 2nd or 3rd. Test yourself doing intervals in a higher heart rate zone by increasing speed or resistance. If you can handle it, start doing that type of interval regularly. If you increase your interval work too slowly, your fitness will not improve further. There is no best schedule for this kind of training. You have to find an optimal progression between over doing it and advancing too slowly.

High intensity effort	Heart rate per effort	Recovery between efforts	Number of efforts per set	Number of sets	Recovery between sets
1 minute	Zone 2	3 minutes	1	1	-
2 minutes	Zone 2	3 minutes	2	2	10 minutes
2 minutes	Zone 3	3 minutes	2	1	-
2 minutes	Zone 3	3 minutes	4	1	-
2 minutes	Zone 3	3 minutes	3	2	10 minutes
4 minutes	Zone 3	5 minutes	3	2	15 minutes
15 seconds	Zone 4	5 minutes	2	1	-
30 seconds	Zone 4	5 minutes	2	2	15 minutes
30 seconds	Zone 4	5 minutes	3	2	15 minutes
1 minute	Zone 4	5 minutes	3	3	20 minutes
8 seconds	Zone 5	5 minutes	3	1	-
8 seconds	Zone 5	5 minutes	3	2	15 minutes
15 seconds	Zone 5	1 minute	5	1	-
1 minute	Zone 5	5 minutes	4	2	20 minutes

Figure 10.6 Examples of high intensity intervals listed from easier to harder.

Intensity of intervals. Intense effort is relative to what is normal for you. If you are a new exerciser or new to the practice of exercising hard, don't push yourself too quickly. Start by doing intervals one zone above the zone your heart rate reaches during your usual exercise. Estimate your heart rate zone using the guidelines in the "Measure Your Exercise Intensity" section. If your routine evening walk is very leisurely, below your aerobic threshold, start with intervals in Zone 2. If you already can exercise into the low aerobic range, try some intervals in Zone 3, the mid-aerobic range. New exercisers should be able to maintain Zone 3 efforts for several minutes or longer. After you become accustomed to these hard efforts, try some intervals in Zone 4. Training in Zone 4 up to the anaerobic threshold has a powerful fitness effect.

Recovery generally should be in Zone 2, the low end of the aerobic range. If you feel very spent after the interval, it is fine to drop down below your aerobic threshold, Zone 1, for a while to feel relieved. If you had been exercising very leisurely, almost all in Zone 1, your recovery level after practicing Zone 2 intervals would be Zone 1.

For the non-competitive athlete and new exerciser, there is no need for Zone 5 training, at least not during the first several months or even year after having started at an unfit level. It can take a long while to adapt to high intensity work. Functionally, maximum physical effort is important in competition, but for the ordinary person who is more concerned about daily function and physical well-being, working up to Zone 4 is adequate. It's enough for a substantial fitness benefit and will produce the psychological gains of adapting to different exercise, creating interest and challenge, and being flexible. If after some time you become inspired to participate in a race or you like to compete with friends on group rides or runs, Zone 5 training will help you cope with intense work and teach your body to perform at its maximum capacity.

Structured versus unstructured intervals. You can make your intervals structured or unstructured. The physical benefit will be the same if the time and intensity are reasonably equivalent, but the psychological experience is very different. Both approaches have advantages for deepening your exercise habit, but in different ways.

Structured intervals. Structured intervals are timed efforts that go strictly by the clock. You increase your heart rate to your target zone, then watch the clock and return to an easier effort when the time is over (Figure 10.6). For example, let's say you are going to do one-minute speed intervals on a bike. After warming up, you come to a flat stretch of road and increase your pedaling speed until you reach the Zone 4 threshold. You pedal consistently at that intensity until one minute elapses, then you ease back on pedaling until your heart rate drops down to Zone 1. You continue easy pedaling for five minutes before starting the next speed increase to Zone 4. All the while, you are watching the time. Indoor cardio machines usually have built-in electronic programs for timed intervals that force speed or working against more resistance.

Following a strict time schedule from a training point of view is important, because if you want to increase your fitness, you will need to gradually increase the amount of time in small increments. To do this, you need an objective, accurate measure – a watch, not your subjective estimate. People are not good estimators of time, especially short intervals of seconds or minutes, and tend to overestimate the elapse of time when engaged in hard work.

Psychologically, exercising by the clock will make you more hardy. By hardy I mean better able to withstand unpleasant or difficult exercise feelings and to resist urges to quit. For example, let's say that

Zone 4 interval feels really intense, so intense you are panting and slobbering, your legs are getting sore, and you're telling yourself "I can't do this; it's too hard." If you have time left on the clock and keep going, you now have had some practice being hardy. That will make it less likely you'll quit the next time you do high intensity intervals. More importantly, you should cope better with real situations when hard work is required.

For instance, you are on vacation and following a walking tour up steep hills. It's hard, really hard, but you have to keep up or miss the tour guide's commentary and maybe lose the group. Having had experience with timed intervals, you are used to walking strenuously further than feels comfortable. Fundamentally, time intervals require you to work in response to an external demand – the clock – rather than an internal demand – your subjective feeling of fatigue and desire to quit. When the control over how much time to exercise is external, you are forced to overcome urges to quit.

Time intervals are especially important for competitive aerobic athletes. At crucial times in a race situation you must increase your effort to stay in the pack or catch a competitor who accelerates away from you. You are forced to follow the other person's pace rather than your own. If during training you always stop when you are tired, you'll be unable to keep going in a race when people around you act like they are not as tired as you. Timed intervals prepare you to respond to external demands to push yourself physically and to cope with discomfort and suffering.

Unstructured intervals. Unstructured intervals do not require a set distance or time. You begin the exercise session planning to do some hard efforts, but exactly when and how long are not dictated by the watch. In fact, you don't even need a watch. You use other cues to inspire you to start an interval. For outside activities such as walking, hiking, running, or cycling, the easiest cues are landmarks on the route ahead of you. When you are warmed-up and ready, look for a tree, driveway, telephone pole, intersection or something else in the distance to which you can pick up the pace and sustain a hard effort. After reaching that place, start the recovery interval. Recovery also is not dictated by the watch. Move ahead at an easy pace until you are breathing easily again and your heart rate has settled down. Continue for a while until feeling rested. Sometime later, visualize another landmark for the next interval. Move fast to that and recover and so on.

You can create unstructured intervals for any type of aerobic exercise. On the water, visualize a target like a landmark on the shore, birds floating on the water, or a mooring. In the gym, pick-up the intensity on the treadmill or elliptical machine during the commercial break on the TV monitor or for the length of a song on your MP3 player.

The principle of working at different intensities or heart rate zones still applies when practicing unstructured intervals. Intervals in the higher zones are shorter. To get a Zone 5 interval, pick a target just 100 yards away and sprint. For someone who recently started high intensity exercise and is working on Zone 3 efforts, find a landmark further away like an intersection one-quarter mile down the road. For the person who has adapted to efforts throughout the aerobic and anaerobic range, mix-up the intervals to cover all the zones. To accumulate the proper amount of high intensity work using an unstructured approach requires some awareness and honesty. There is no clock to judge you, so a program of just unstructured work is risky. On the other hand, there are great psychological and practical advantages of unstructured intervals.

The origin of unstructured high intensity work is "fartlek", a

Swedish training technique, translated as "speed play". The term speaks for an important advantage of this approach – play. It's a lot more playful and fun to do your intervals spontaneously when the urge or opportunity arises. It's a lot more fun to mix it up with different intensities instead of repeating the same thing over and over by the clock. High intensity exercise is hard work. Speed play allows you to be creative and spontaneous.

Not having an exact plan for intervals allows you to change exercise intensity as needed. You can listen to your body instead of the clock. If you have no trouble getting into your heart rate zone, then go ahead and do your high intensity work. If your heart rate isn't getting into the zone it should given your effort or you're having a hard time working hard, you probably are not rested enough. Reduce your work to a lower intensity interval. An unstructured approach lets you change as the need arises. In contrast, when doing structured intervals, athletes who have trouble getting into zone usually will cancel the high intensity workout altogether, because that is an all or nothing approach. Speed play is dynamic and adaptive.

You also can adapt more easily to the terrain and people around you. If you are in hilly terrain, it will be hard to do only leg speed intervals. With an unstructured approach, you can do strength, high resistance intervals uphill and mix it up with some leg speed intervals on the downhill run-out. Groups of recreational exercisers, like walking groups, cycling clubs and so forth, are out for recreation – fun, rather than a rigid clock driven workout. Although it can be done, telling your friends "Excuse me, I need to get a couple 120 second Zone 5 intervals" can be awkward and unsocial. Instead, you can incorporate occasional bursts of hard efforts when they fit into the rhythm of the group, such as a hard hill climb when the group normally stretches out anyway with strong climbers at the front. Unstructured high intensity work helps strengthen your habit by making exercise more fun and adaptive.

Controlling self-talk. High intensity intervals are meant to be hard and to stress your body. The challenge is to make it through the exercise without quitting or suffering more than necessary. This is determined a great deal by how you talk to yourself. Unlike easier low intensity exercise that you do without much thinking, for high intensity exercise you will have to talk yourself into doing it. During the intervals beware that the more preoccupied you are with suffering, the more suffering you will feel. If you start thinking of excuses to stop, you will be more likely to quit. Focusing on negative experiences and urges to escape will create the outcome you wish to avoid.

After a high intensity workout, it's normal to feel spent and pained, to think, "I'll never do that again." Our early ancestors needed to push themselves to their physical limits in order to survive and to repeat painful bursts of physical activity again and again. To cope, there must have been some selective amnesia for the pain of intense exercise. This helpful psychological trick probably became encoded in human nature, because now we know exercisers who plan another hard workout seem to forget or downplay how much it hurt last time. But forgetting the pain of exercise depends a lot on you.

Fortunately, you have the power to control your mental reaction by practicing helpful self-talk. Rational self-talk about how good you will feel after accomplishing your workout, distraction techniques to focus on other sensations or thoughts, reframing physical symptoms as positive experiences, thoughts of mastering a challenge, thoughts of competence and self-efficacy, and confidence in finishing your workout – these self-talk strategies will help you finish your workout and to avoid overly negative memories. If it's hard to think when you're working out hard, try music or podcasts. They can mask unpleasant sounds of heavy breathing and keep negative thoughts out of your head.

Medium, fun days. Medium, fun days are just that: medium and fun. They are a break from the concentration and effort of high intensity intervals and long endurance workouts. On those hard days, you push yourself physically and psychologically. On the medium days you exercise energetically, but not to the point of fatigue. If you did intervals and hard efforts every day, if you always had to exercise exactly by the clock, you would start feeling burned out, stressed, and tired. But cycling between those hard and medium efforts creates fitness, better than if you went hard all the time. If you have reached four days per week of exercise but have not started endurance or high intensity days, medium intensity exercise should be your normal type of workout.

On medium fun days, exercise feels more like recreation and less like work or medicine. Now it's time to enjoy yourself. You worked hard. Now you feel strong and confident. It's fun to enjoy that, to appreciate your fitness and accomplishment. It's time just to be physical and to play and not to worry about being ambitious. When your hard work is rewarded with relief, it is easier to face the next bout of hard exercise.

Intensity and length of medium exercise. Good for your recovery, medium days aren't completely easy going either. Medium intensity ideally is in the low to medium aerobic range, Zones 2-3. It is an exercise intensity that you can continue for a long while without feeling exhausted or sore. This is the same intensity level as you should target for your endurance day. The difference is the length of exercise time. As is the case for the other types of exercise days, the specific heart rate for medium is relative to where your fitness is at the present time.

If you are able to do high intensity intervals in Zone 4 or Zone 5, your medium days can be Zones 2 and 3. If Zone 3 is high intensity for you now, keep your heart rate in Zone 2 as much as possible, with some time spent in Zone 1 being okay as well. If you just started some time working in the low aerobic range, Zone 2, then a normal medium day is probably mainly Zone 1. If this latter example describes you, be sure to continue one, preferably two, days of high intensity intervals in order to improve your aerobic capacity. Be patient and persistent. After some weeks of intervals and a greater overall number of hours exercise per week, you should feel comfortable keeping your heart rate in Zone 2 for a full exercise episode.

There is no rigid standard for length of a medium workout, other than it is less, at least 50 percent less than an endurance workout. The example in Figure 10.5 shows medium days more and less than high intensity days. Since the emphasis is on having fun, the only time issue is to add enough medium exercise time in order to make your overall goal for total time for the week.

When to do medium days. There is no single best order of exercise intensity. The example in Figure 10.5 shows the more challenging days of high intensity and endurance alternating with medium, fun days. That approach lets you anticipate some relief the day after working hard. It's certainly reasonable to do all your hard days in a row, preferably with an endurance day in-between the two high intensity days in order to allow some recovery from intervals. The best order might be determined by circumstances such as work schedule or weather. In particular, it can be difficult to do an endurance episode if you are tight for time or the weather for outdoor activities is unfavorable. Sticking to a standard weekly plan helps to make varying exercise intensity a habit, because you do not have to make decisions about what to do each day. "Tuesday and Thursday are my short, hard days. Saturday is my long day." An engrained expectation like that makes it easier to say "No" to other temptations. On the other hand, being flexible makes you adaptable so you reorganize your schedule when facing unusual circumstances. Plus, being spontaneous can be fun.

Medium does not mean sitting on the couch. It means repeating the same physical activity but at a lower intensity, an intensity at which you can smell the roses a little more. Unlike an interval day when you might find a hill and repeat climbing it over and over for your intensity intervals, a medium day is going where you want without overly structuring it. To have fun while maintaining fitness is your goal.

Recovery day. Stressing the body with intense exercise leads to breakdown of your muscle and other soft tissue, depletion of your energy stores, and build-up of waste byproducts that can make you feel sore and tired. You adapt to the stress and become more physically fit if you allow yourself a rest period. During rest time, your energy is replenished and your body repairs itself. You return from rest stronger and better able to handle the next bout of hard work. If you do not cycle between hard and easy work, recovery from intense exercise will be incomplete. You will feel tired and unable to keep going hard and your fitness – the capacity to do physical work – will actually go down. Depletion of energy can make you feel ill and the continual breakdown of muscle and connective tissue can lead to injury. Psychologically, you will feel stale during exercise – a sort of disinterest and loss of enthusiasm. You won't feel frisky or peppy. You won't be the only stressed person. People around you might be offended if you do not take time off. Many people assume that to become physically fit, exercise has to be intense every time – otherwise it's not exercise. But a recovery day

IS exercise, a form of rest that allows you to adapt and become stronger.

Recovery workouts are for people who are exercising at least four days per week and are spending much of their exercise time in the aerobic range. If you haven't achieved this level yet, work on increasing your exercise frequency and add some interval or endurance training to your repertoire.

Intensity and length of recovery exercise. A recovery day should not be a day of sitting and resting on the couch. The best recovery is active recovery. In the Tour de France, the bicycle racers have a couple rest days during the three weeks of riding over 100 miles, day after day. What do these men do on their day off? Ride their bikes! Yes, the best way to repair your body, to remove waste products from strenuous exercise is to repeat the same activity at an easy intensity. Work the same muscles that you use for endurance or high intensity workouts, but for just a short time without much muscular effort.

If you are a walker and hiker, it's best to recover with a short easy walk rather than to take the day off completely. If you are a cyclist, it's best to do an easy ride. An easy day of kayaking after days of hiking might feel restful and be a good mental break, but will not be as helpful physically, because completely different muscles and motions are used.

There is no firm guideline for the length of recovery exercise. Move long enough to feel awake and somewhat energetic. If you're sore from the previous day, move until some of the soreness dissipates. The example in Figure 10.5 shows a recovery day about one-third of a normal, medium day. More or less is fine as well, so long as you avoid approaching the length of an endurance workout.

Recovery exercise is below the aerobic threshold - strictly in Zone 1. Zone 1 IS exercise. Sitting on the couch is "zone 0". That's not a good way to repair the body from a good week of exercise. To keep your heart rate in Zone 1, choose a workout that will not require hard work. Walking or riding flat terrain instead of hills will help. Put your bicycle gear into the small chain ring and pedal easily. Keep the treadmill flat, at a slower speed. Lower the resistance on the elliptical machine. By reducing the speed or strength required for your normal workout, your heart rate should be lower. To be sure, check yourself repeatedly as you exercise. If your heart rate goes into Zone 2 or higher, cut back on the intensity until your heart rate is in Zone 1.

Coping with recovery. Psychologically, recovery can be a challenge because taking it easy for a day defies the image of exercise as sweat and hard work. When progressing on the development of an exercise habit, it's normal to fear slipping back into a sedentary lifestyle. Easy exercise outings can be mistakenly equated with acting slothful again. Even athletes, who know that rest is important for optimal performance, can feel guilty or worried about taking it easy. Consequently, it's not uncommon for people to overdo it and end up hurting rather than improving their fitness. Recovering requires that you resist temptation to exercise hard every day. Put the recovery day on your calendar and stick to it. Monitor your heart rate. If you are going too hard, interrupt yourself. Use appropriate self-talk. Tell yourself to slow down. Reassure yourself that you ARE exercising, that doing an easy workout is good for you.

Take advantage of your recovery days to do something different and easy. For instance, bike riding with my wife is a recovery day for me and the bonus is, I can ride at her pace and know I'm accomplishing something. Or I might use a recovery day to ride or hike with my young grandchildren. It's a perfect way to move, but not stress myself.

Overdoing it is one problem. Another trap is skipping exercise altogether on what should be a recovery day. The reasoning is something like this: "If I'm not going to get a good workout, why bother doing anything"; "An easy stroll around the neighborhood doesn't feel like exercise, I'll wait until tomorrow and do my normal walk." This is all-or-nothing thinking; black-and-white thinking that denies the value of a recovery workout because it's beneath your capacity. But the opposite of hard exercise - sitting on the couch - does not help your fitness either. It's not recovery. Correct self-talk that says it's okay to skip an active recovery session. Remind yourself that to recover will help you feel rested and stronger.

If you exercise with friends, fitting recovery with their pace takes some determination and creativity. Be strict with yourself. Don't let other people who are moving faster sweep you into a higher heart rate zone. Keep it slow and true to your fitness. Among athletes in training, it's perfectly normal to announce "I'm having a recovery day and taking it easy." Ask others to wait for you at the top of a hill if you are trying to climb at a low heart rate. Stay at the back of the group with the slower walkers. Cut the day short by returning early so you do not walk or ride too long. Skip the group for the day if their plan is to do something harder than you should.

When to do a recovery day. Recovery should happen after a stretch of intense exercise. For instance, Monday might be a good day for people who are limited to the weekend for big physical activity. But if you can't do a recovery day exactly after your intense days, don't worry. Do it when it fits your schedule. You will help your fitness, all the same. I have argued that to deepen your exercise habit, to make you resistant to relapsing back to being a non-exerciser, it's important to become flexible and adaptive. That way, any day regardless of circumstances can be an exercise day. Use the need to recover to fit exercise into odd days when it's hard to exercise normally. If real busy, get away for a quick easy swim or walk. Do it then, when you don't have enough time to squeeze in a long workout. If you're travelling, take advantage of circumstances and walk the airport terminal for recovery. Try walking or riding to the market or to some other errand in town for an easy outing. Maybe the family is doing something easy like beachcombing that would be a good Zone 1 outing for you – and would double as quality time with others.

Ultimately, when to recover should be determined by your state of fitness rather than the calendar. Let's say you did not schedule a recovery workout today, but you had trouble getting to a higher heart rate zone. Instead of pressing on with hard work, you should listen to your body. Inability to raise your heart rate or feeling tired at your normal exercise level is a symptom of not being rested. Pushing yourself to do a workout your body does not want will make you more tired rather than stronger. It's time to revise your plan on the fly and work on recovery instead.

Variety Is Good For Habit

Regardless of how important physical fitness is to prevent disease and slow the aging process, the immediate benefit is that exercise will feel much easier and less tiring. And as a result you will want to exercise more. One of the best ways to improve physical fitness is to add variety to your exercise intensity on a regular basis, including bouts of endurance and higher intensity exercise. Psychologically, you will be more flexible and adaptive to circumstances if you have learned how to exercise at the different levels of intensity. And as a result you are less likely to have an exercise lapse.

To vary exercise intensity in a systematic way requires ramping up dedication and commitment to your fitness. Harder workouts, more time, and more careful measurement. If all this sounds like too much, simply start with the basic – measure your exercise intensity every day and write it in your diary. Don't force any further change. Self-monitoring will work its magic and soon motivate you to start controlling exercise intensity. Enjoy.

Chapter 11: Become Hardy

Exercise is supposed to feel good, but if it were totally positive and satisfying, most people would not struggle to make exercise a habit. Bad weather, social pressure to not exercise, and intense, unpleasant, even scary physical sensations. No wonder exercise can be a hardship rather than joy. Adversity is almost an inseparable part of exercise. Even people with strong incentives to work hard on their fitness like competitive athletes and people in physical rehabilitation must overcome negative experiences and suffering before they succeed. The ability to face exercise challenges, to endure, and frankly, to suffer separate the winners from the losers, the consistent exercisers from the quitters. This chapter will help you understand how to make yourself more hardy. To start, it's necessary to understand how people learn to not be hardy – to avoid, rather than to face adversity – and why avoidance is so harmful to an exercise habit.

Avoidance And Giving Up – The Basics

One of the easiest behavioral responses to learn is to avoid something that is frightening or harmful. It's easy because avoidance is adaptive. Early human beings depended on being able to flee danger and to avoid aversive experiences in order to survive. Although modern civilization protects people from most life-threatening dangers that were faced by our ancestors, there still are plenty of uncomfortable experiences in daily life that can trigger the urge to avoid. Avoidance is deeply engrained biologically in our behavioral repertoire. But avoidance to specific situations can be learned and if we so desire, unlearned.

An easy way to understand how avoidance can be learned is to consider the anxiety problem in a phobia. Let's say dogs frighten you because one as a child attacked you. As an adult, you still feel anxious whenever you encounter a dog regardless of how friendly it really might be. You feel anxious and want to get out of the situation. After escaping, you feel relieved. Because the feeling of anxiety is so intense and negative, relief is a powerful reward for the escape behavior. Over time, escaping or avoidance becomes a strong behavior – it's been rewarded by anxiety reduction. In a way, it feels good to give-up. See the diagram in Figure 11.1. The direction of the arrows indicates that feelings of relief encourage avoidance. The table in Figure 11.1 shows how this applies to the example of fear of dogs.

Avoidance and escape are similar coping mechanisms, but refer to different points in time in the process of dealing with anxiety. To avoid means to not expose yourself to the aversive experience at all, such as to not go to a place where you suspect there might be a dog. Anticipation of a dangerous dog triggers anxiety. Avoidance provides relief. Whereas escape refers to getting away from an aversive stimulus. Exposure to a dog that you perceive as dangerous triggers anxiety. Escape provides relief. For the sake of this discussion, I'll use the two terms interchangeably.

Escape and avoidance are protective mechanisms and provide immediate relief, but in the long run, they create unintended problems that perpetuate discomfort. Ironically, a fear response will become stronger the more you avoid the scary or difficult situation. One reason is that you do not have any experience facing and coping with the anxiety. You've blocked it by avoidance. That prevents you from learning how to tolerate anxiety. Moreover, you do not learn that the situation is not as dangerous as you imagined. You do not accumulate evidence to prove that some or all of your fear was irrational. Using the fear of dogs example: if you never let yourself be around a dog, you wouldn't understand that under normal circumstances, dogs like people and do not attack strangers. And you wouldn't learn to discriminate truly dangerous dog situations. If you never forced yourself to face a scary dog situation, you wouldn't learn how to be calmer around dogs.

Behavior always occurs in a chain of responses. A reward for one behavior can encourage the behaviors that precede it. So, if anxiety reduction rewards avoidance behavior, it will reward the response that precedes the avoidance as well. In this case, the response earlier in the chain is the anxiety itself: feeling anxious, acting anxious, thinking in an anxious manner – all these are rewarded along with the avoidance behavior that is intended to eliminate anxiety in the first instance. Look again at the diagram in Figure 11.1 to see how these processes affect one another. The arrows show the chain of responses and the backward influence of reward. Relief rewards avoidance or escape and going further back along the behavior chain, relief also rewards the experience of adversity itself.

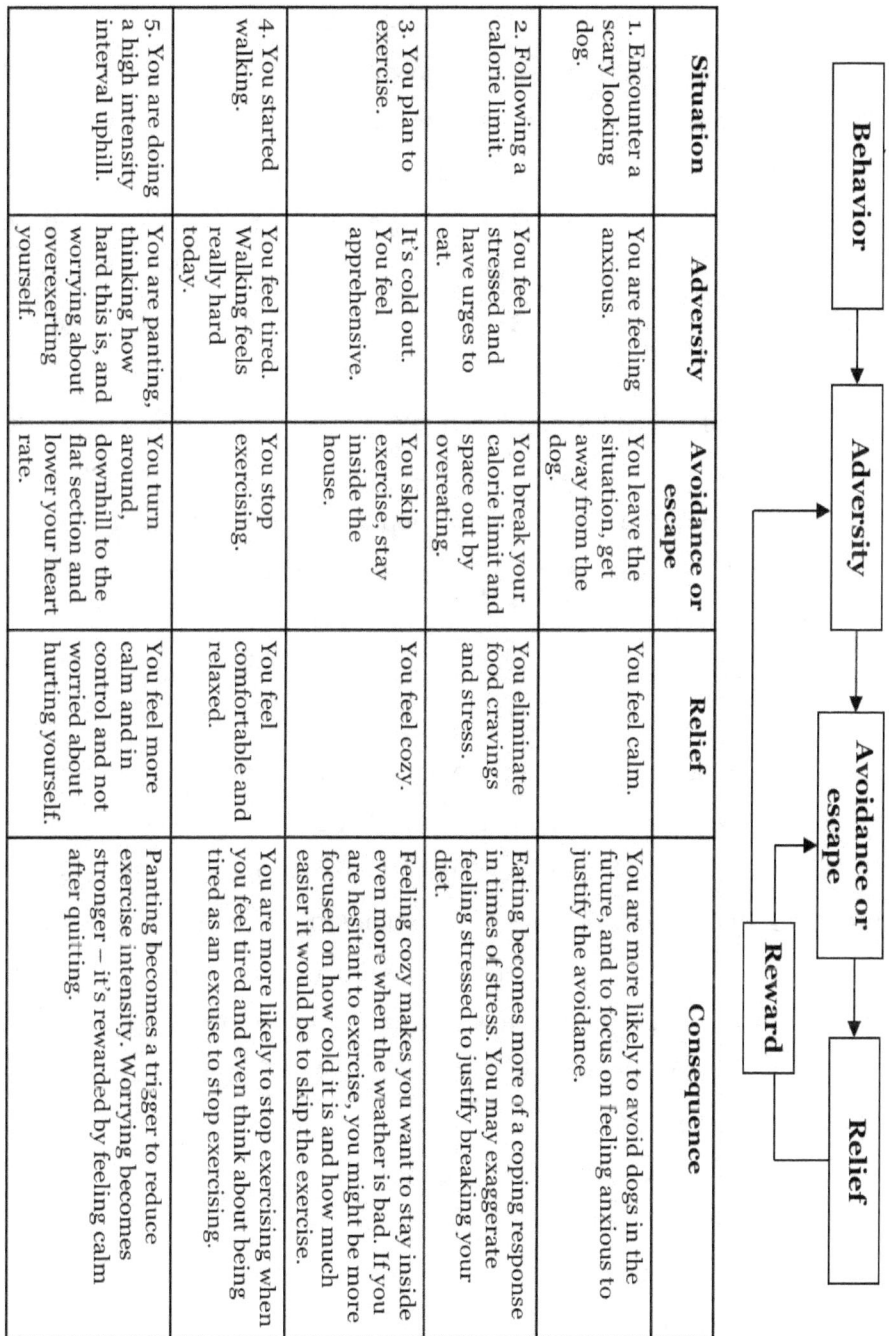

Situation	Adversity	Avoidance or escape	Relief	Consequence
1. Encounter a scary looking dog.	You are feeling anxious.	You leave the situation, get away from the dog.	You feel calm.	You are more likely to avoid dogs in the future, and to focus on feeling anxious to justify the avoidance.
2. Following a calorie limit.	You feel stressed and have urges to eat.	You break your calorie limit and space out by overeating.	You eliminate food cravings and stress.	Eating becomes more of a coping response in times of stress. You may exaggerate feeling stressed to justify breaking your diet.
3. You plan to exercise.	It's cold out. You feel apprehensive.	You skip exercise, stay inside the house.	You feel cozy.	Feeling cozy makes you want to stay inside even more when the weather is bad. If you are hesitant to exercise, you might be more focused on how cold it is and how much easier it would be to skip the exercise.
4. You started walking.	You feel tired. Walking feels really hard today.	You stop exercising.	You feel comfortable and relaxed.	You are more likely to stop exercising when you feel tired and even think about being tired as an excuse to stop exercising.
5. You are doing a high intensity interval uphill.	You are panting, thinking how hard this is, and worrying about overexerting yourself.	You turn around, downhill to the flat section and lower your heart rate.	You feel more calm and in control and not worried about hurting yourself.	Panting becomes a trigger to reduce exercise intensity. Worrying becomes stronger – it's rewarded by feeling calm after quitting.

Behavior → Adversity → Avoidance or escape → Relief

Reward

Figure 11.1. Relief from adversity encourages avoidance and giving up.

The second example, overeating under stress, shows how this very subtle process occurs. You are trying to control your weight and stick to a calorie limit. A time comes when you feel stressed. Your way to cope with this adversity is to escape by overeating – it's comforting to overeat, to indulge yourself, and to space out with food. That escape mechanism helps eliminate feeling stressed – overeating is rewarded. What are the consequences? The most obvious one is overeating might become a habit because it helps you control stress. The other is very subtle: you might feel more stress in the future. Why? Well, if it feels so good to overeat, you might become even more attentive to sensations of stress, you might think more about stress in order to justify overeating. In a way, feeling stressed could magnify and become an excuse to overeat.

To face feelings or to run away from them is a coping style that is influenced by culture and family. Generally, people value being strong and able to face up to life's challenges. To excuse oneself, to escape can be a threat to self-esteem. We don't want to admit we are making ourselves feel worse just so we can indulge ourselves or escape into a stupor. Therefore, this process of making adversity more adverse in order to get the rewarding consequence of relief usually is subconscious or out of awareness. Regardless of how aware you might be, habitually giving-up in the face of adversity will make you feel more bothered in the future.

Avoidance And Giving-Up Exercise

There are plenty of unpleasant experiences in exercise to avoid. Let's look at Figure 11.1 again to consider some typical examples of exercise adversity and the effect of avoidance.

Bad weather, such as very cold temperature, makes it more challenging for people who exercise outdoors. As a transplant from

California, the sometimes-frigid winter conditions in Vermont were shocking. But I learned to cope with the cold by getting into winter sports and wearing the right clothes. It was amusing that many native Vermonters with lifelong winter experience stayed indoors and surrendered physical activity when it was really cold. Besides missing out on a lot of fun, that was a recipe for a weak exercise habit.

But staying inside on cold or bad weather days is really easy to learn (Example 3). Being in cold air can trigger breathing problems. Sweaty clothes can freeze and cause a loss of body heat. The hands and face can feel chilled or numb. Rain or snow soaking through clothes is unpleasant. Thoughts of catching a cold can be worrisome. Wearing extra layers can make normal exercise less fun. Just getting dressed with all the right clothes can be a hassle. It's a lot simpler to skip all this and go with the cozy feeling and look at the outside from inside your warm home. Those feelings of relief will encourage you to keep avoiding cold weather and prevent you from learning how to deal with it or to discover that the cold isn't so bad after all. If it's terribly unpleasant outside, of course, it is reasonable to find an alternative exercise. On the other hand, most people who struggle with an exercise habit frankly would rather not exercise when they have a good excuse. Going backward up the chain of responses, if you start dwelling on how bad it might feel out in the cold, you'll want to avoid it as well as exercise. Ultimately the more focused on the cold and feeling apprehensive, the better your excuse to avoid it.

How often do you skip exercise like in Example 4? After a long day of work, it's difficult to motivate yourself to work on your fitness. Who wants to work hard exercising after a hard day at work? It's normal to want to space out and relax instead of getting dressed and going for a nice hardy walk. Although exercise might be a good way to wake-up and reduce stress, you would have to break through those initial feelings of fatigue in order to keep going. That takes some mental concentration on how good you might feel after. But often the mind automatically tries to support the temptation to escape, because that offers immediate gratification and no effort. Comfort and relaxation are rewards for skipping that walk. Subconsciously, to justify escape, you must dwell on how tired you feel instead of the good things that might happen if you kept going. The positive consequences of escaping encourage dwelling on negative thoughts. Feeling fatigue and thinking about it becomes a learned trigger for not exercising.

High intensity exercise is hard even under the best of circumstances and at the beginning it can feel utterly painful and scary. Example 5 diagrams relief after quitting an interval. If you feel panicked about panting and overexertion but escape, you would not learn it's safe and manageable to finish. That relief will be especially powerful because the worrisome feelings were so intense. Quitting becomes a strong escape behavior and in the future, you might be tempted to dwell on the bad feelings in order to justify quitting.

Learn To Be Hardy

To be hardy means to be capable of withstanding adverse conditions. You learn to be hardy by facing adversity over and over again. In time, you tolerate adversity. You are not as bothered. You even look forward to it because good feelings of pride and strength are your reward. Learning to be hardy is difficult, not because people are weak or the adversity is so unpleasant, but because people who struggle with exercise tend to practice exercise when conditions are favorable and otherwise skip it. To become hardy requires facing up to difficult circumstances when they arise and even intentionally finding adversity to become more hardy. The longer-term rewards for exercise hardiness are improved health, fitness, weight loss and a stronger exercise habit. Being hardy makes your exercise habit stronger because you impose fewer limitations on when or how to exercise. Enduring more difficult exercise makes you stronger physically which rewards your effort and makes exercise more fun.

The diagram in Figure 11.2 shows this process. The payoffs for being hardy are the good feelings and fitness that result, plus, going backward in the behavior chain, the experience of adversity itself. Yes, over time, it can feel good to put yourself in a situation that feels hard, because such challenges result in great feelings of accomplishment after.

3. You are timing 4 minute high intensity intervals on the treadmill.	Your legs are sore and you feel like it's too hard to keep going, but the clock hasn't reached 4 minutes.	You distract yourself from negative self-talk and continue to the stop time on the first. clock.	Wow. It feels great to have done intervals that seemed too hard at first.	You feel more confident about high intensity workouts, less likely to think of quitting, and even look forward to the hard days.
4. Your walking partner is not available. You have to walk alone.	It's boring and you feel self-conscious.	You do your usual walk anyway.	You are proud of sticking to your schedule and being more independent.	Walking alone is no longer as unpleasant. You enjoy being flexible.
5. Trying something new – a spinning class.	You feel like a klutz and wonder how you look to other people.	You keep telling yourself "I have a right to be here."	The workout felt great. You are proud of getting outside of your comfort zone.	You are more likely to do spinning in the future. Trying new things in front of more experienced people becomes a positive challenge.

Figure 11.2. Hardiness is encouraged by feelings of accomplishment, pride and fitness.

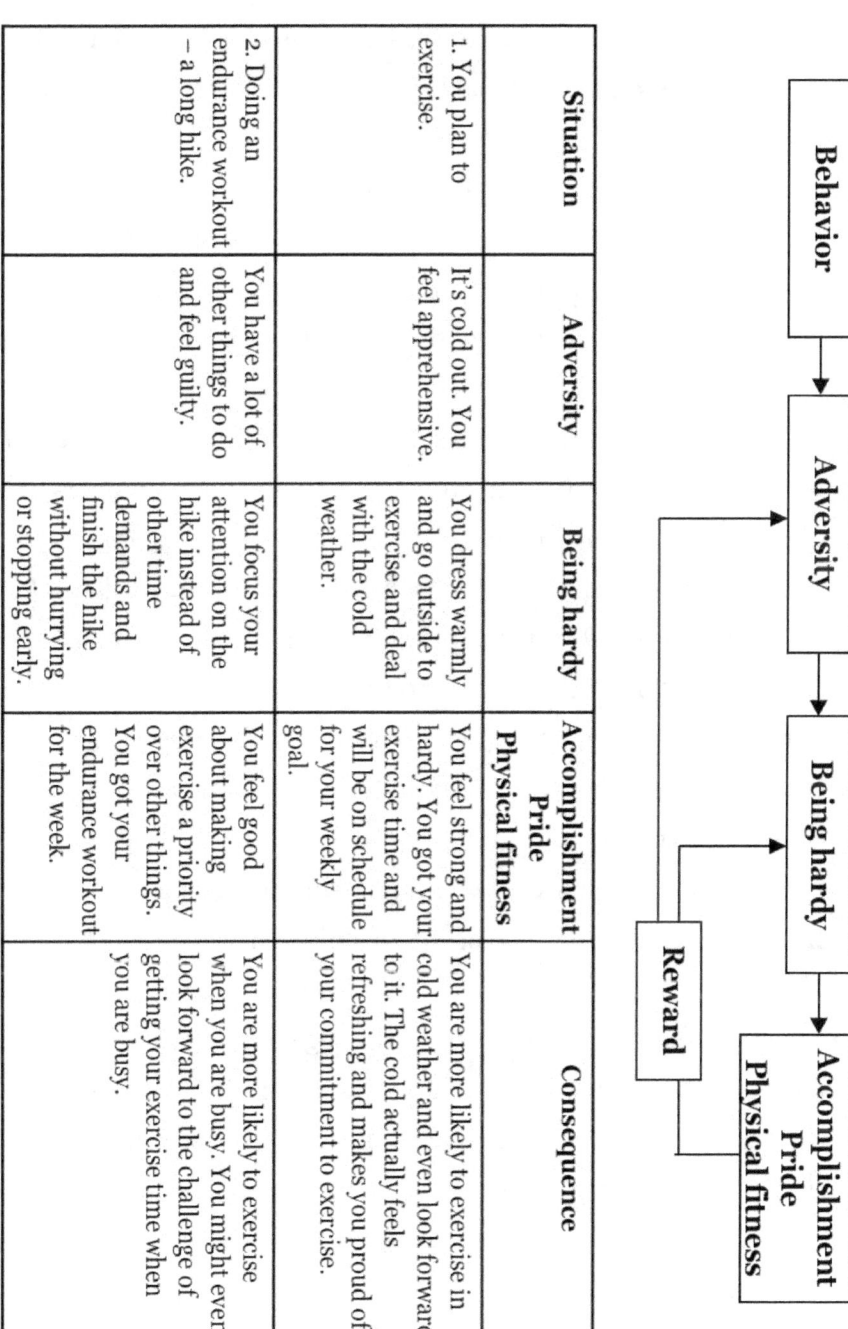

Situation	Adversity	Being hardy	Accomplishment Pride Physical fitness	Consequence
1. You plan to exercise.	It's cold out. You feel apprehensive.	You dress warmly and go outside to exercise and deal with the cold weather.	You feel strong and hardy. You got your exercise time and will be on schedule for your weekly goal.	You are more likely to exercise in cold weather and even look forward to it. The cold actually feels refreshing and makes you proud of your commitment to exercise.
2. Doing an endurance workout – a long hike.	You have a lot of other things to do and feel guilty.	You focus your attention on the hike instead of other time demands and finish the hike without hurrying or stopping early.	You feel good about making exercise a priority over other things. You got your endurance workout for the week.	You are more likely to exercise when you are busy. You might even look forward to the challenge of getting your exercise time when you are busy.

Behavior → Adversity → Being hardy → Accomplishment Pride Physical fitness

Reward

Exercise hardiness. All the examples of hardiness in Figure 11.2 involve persisting under circumstances that feel unpleasant or stressful. Among other consequences, the most important is that acting hardy helped the exerciser actually do the exercise that was planned, as opposed to give-up or avoid it. Sticking to an exercise schedule is what it takes to become more fit and to deepen your exercise habit. Being hardy means overcoming temptation, excuses, and adversity to make it happen.

Can you relate to any of these? How about Example 1 – dressing up for the cold weather and despite the temptation to stay indoors, you felt proud for not letting the cold keep you from exercising. Maybe you even felt refreshed by the cold and look forward to trying it again.

A great way to become more hardy and to tolerate intense workouts is to follow the clock instead of quitting when you are tired or suffering. In Example 3, it took mental control to resist urges to quit the 4-minute interval. With continued practice, interval training should become more tolerable.

To deal with cold weather and suffering during intervals are two examples of being hardy in response to physical adversity. Exercise presents plenty of psychological and social adversity as well. Examples 2, 4, and 5 are stresses that commonly trigger avoidance of exercise: guilt about taking time from other responsibilities, not having an exercise partner, and feeling awkward in front of other people. Acting hardy in these situations can turn busy times, being alone, or trying something new into positive rather than aversive experiences – because making it through them boosts your confidence. Eventually you enjoy being challenged just for the opportunity to test yourself and to conquer your weaker tendency.

Planned hardiness. If you like to challenge and toughen

yourself, you can go out of your way to practice being hardy. Liberate yourself from unhelpful limitations on your exercise.

Let's say it's going to be a cold morning and warm afternoon. You're squeamish about exercising in the cold, but decide to do your walk in the morning anyway, simply to desensitize yourself to cold weather. Or what if your walking partner can't do the morning walk and wants to reschedule for the evening? You could reschedule, but you decide to walk alone at the normal time to help you cope with not having an exercise buddy. Or you are supposed to do a long bike ride today for endurance training. Your endurance rides are getting longer, but feeling tired or worrying about work makes you stop too soon. Today you set a time limit and keep going until the clock says stop.

To overcome a more serious inhibition, gradually face the difficult experience, step by step. Let's use an example of a body image concern that bothered my client's exercise. She felt overly self-conscious about her weight, especially her fat arms. That's why she wore long sleeve sweatshirts on the gym treadmill. But hiding her arms with heavy clothing made her overheated. Her dream was to wear a sleeveless top, but doing that all at once would have been intolerable. So, she began by working out with her sleeves rolled up. When reasonably comfortable with that, she wore short sleeves. And then she switched to sleeveless, at first when no one else in the cardio room and finally when it was busy with other people.

The method is, "expose" yourself to the anxiety provoking cues and then refrain from escaping. Instead, allow yourself to experience the feelings and use a more helpful way to cope with them. After repeated practice, the formerly feared behavior or situation will seem natural.

It's possible to have a hardiness breakthrough in one trial if you set up your challenge as a test of some negative prediction that hopefully will be disconfirmed. Let's say you try an aerobics class. When you walk in, you feel embarrassed because you're the biggest person. You think (predict), "I can't handle this. I'll panic and people will start looking at me." Tempted to leave, you stayed and used your best coping possible and survived the session. That proved that you might feel self-conscious, but nothing terrible will happen. Your feared outcome was untrue. The situation is more manageable than you thought.

Enjoy Being Hardier

Very active, physically fit people enjoy a little bit of suffering. Admittedly, it's an acquired passion, but normal for many, many people. Try to think of challenging situations as opportunities to grow and be more flexible with exercise, rather than as obstacles that you cannot overcome. It takes some courage to face adversity. Start by dealing with the situations that hold you back from following my recommendations for increasing your frequency, time, and intensity of exercise. Enjoy.

Chapter 12:
Vary Your Type of Exercise

Your assignment is to add some other type of exercise. Exercise can be grouped by the bodily function or the physical skill that is used to perform the exercise, such as aerobic versus muscle strengthening. Indoor versus outdoor activity, urban versus nature, team versus individual sports, ball sports versus human powered activities also are different groupings of exercise. Diverse exercise creates more fitness and protection against disease and injury. Exercise is more fun and challenging with a greater variety of activities. Adding more forms of physical activity not only is good physically and psychologically, but it makes an exercise habit stronger.

Are You Ready To Try Different Types Of Exercise?

The recommendation in this chapter is that you add at least a second physical activity. If you already have a second, then it's time to add a third. You are ready if you are exercising regularly and include some variety to your exercise intensity. Roughly, that means doing some physical activity three to four days a week and in addition to easy or medium days, including one endurance or high intensity workout. No matter how comfortable you may be with your current routine, if you are practicing just one type of activity, adding a second is the next important step.

If you are not at this stage and you are still working on basic increases in exercise, it usually is best to stick with a familiar activity instead of trying something completely different. You might need to return to the self-management skills in previous chapters to progress on your exercise frequency and intensity first.

I'm contradicting myself, but if you are completely stuck and not increasing your exercise time, to add something new right now might be a solution. Assuming it is added and you do not subtract from what you are presently doing, that second activity by itself would boost your weekly total time.

Some people actually do not know what is exercise and need suggestions. Go ahead and read this chapter and find tips for activities that you can do now and would enjoy.

Why Increase Your Exercise Choices?

Learn new exercise situations. A well-rounded exercise routine will expose you to different situations. For instance, say you swim for upper body exercise. For the lower body, you are bicycling. For flexibility, you belong to a yoga class. This combination varies your fitness training, but also takes place in different locations, uses different equipment and clothing, and is practiced with different people. The stimuli associated with exercise multiply with each new activity in your repertoire. More exercise cues predict more exercise behavior.

Be prepared for different physical demands. The specific body part or function that you exercise is the part that develops more fitness. This effect is known as the Specificity Principle in the field of exercise and sports science. So, if you are a walker, your lower body muscles, connective tissue, and joints are being exercised. That means you should be able to handle other demands that resemble walking or use those body parts. However, walking does not prepare you for upper body demands. If you spend a day weeding your garden, you are likely to be more tired and sore than someone whose upper body has been conditioned by kayaking. The more body parts and functions you exercise, the more prepared you will be for different physical demands in not only recreation, but in daily life. This can be called functional fitness; fitness for real life daily activities created by doing exercise that transfers to them. Not exercise for the sake of exercise.

Here are some examples of different types of exercise and being prepared for different physical demands.

You gardened the whole day. Good thing you started working out with weights on top of your walking habit. You're feeling much less pooped than normal.
All you used to do was yoga and weight training, but you're going on a vacation and need to start a walking program. At the moment, you're having trouble walking hills, but practice will eventually help you feel less tired.
You and your wife switched from walking the neighborhood to hiking in the park. Your wife had trouble with the rocky sections of trail. It seemed your balance was better – you attributed that to spending a lot of time walking on rocks while stream fishing.
You want to try skiing again. You aren't worried about having the endurance – you've been cycling a lot. But you want to strengthen the legs to protect the knees.
You were worried about trying snowshoeing with friends. That would involve using poles and shoeing up and down hills. It turned out that you did fine. Maybe those elliptical machine workouts with the ski handles had given you the arm and leg strength you needed.

Add fun and interest to exercise. It's normal to stick with one activity at the beginning in order to start a routine and to get used to exercising more. Eventually, you risk losing interest or feeling burned out if that one activity is all you do. There are so many choices out there. Why not expand your enjoyment by adding some variety.

Find other activities that are amusing, pleasant, stimulating, refreshing, relaxing, and a diversion from routine life. Try one thing new and the next time it will be easier to try another.

Here are some examples of adding interest and fun with new types of activity.

Bicycling is giving you a feeling of freedom. Compared to walking, in the same amount of time you're seeing much more. It's exciting to go a long distance under your own power. And the speed on the bike is refreshing.
You started waterskiing again. That took some nerve, but what a great option to swim and play in a lake instead of the backyard pool. The upper body workout is a bonus.
You like walking but your local routes have become too familiar. You also enjoy fishing and switched from lake to stream fishing as a way to walk, but in nature where you have other distractions to pass the time.
You love golf and your wife loves tennis, but you aren't enjoying any exercise together. It turned out that riding a tandem bicycle was a chance for a different kind of workout and at the same time a pleasant way to be together and talk.
You have been doing calisthenics and aerobic exercise with television in home. Now that you're feeling more confident, you tried an aerobics class at the fitness center. It was intimidating at first, but being in a group was motivating and pushed you to work harder.

Be flexible. Two common reasons people stop exercising, at least temporarily, are suffering an injury and being away from home.

Too many of my clients built-up a large amount of walking time and then, from overuse, developed a foot injury that suspended their walking. That was their sole activity and they had nothing else to fall back on.

Another risk factor for slips, being away from home, is a problem for people who do not have a transportable exercise routine. Getting into cycling is great for your fitness, but you probably would not take your bike on a vacation or business trip.

Having other choices could solve both of these problems. If you can't ride your bike on vacation, how about exercise walks or the fitness center at the hotel. If you can't walk due to a foot injury, how about swimming, cycling, or weight training – something that won't stress the foot. The critical factor for a long-term exercise habit is to minimize disruptions and lapses. Flexible exercise options will help you persist during unusual circumstances.

Check these examples of being flexible in typical risk situations.

You broke your wrist skiing and your main worry was not being able to keep up your cycling. You never thought of walking as worthwhile exercise, but gave it a try. Long hilly walks turned out to be a good workout and helped you cope with the wrist healing. Your solution was to exercise the part of your body that worked.
You've gotten into a good weight training routine, but you're going on vacation. For an aerobic workout, you still can get some decent walking on the golf course. For weight training, you did pushups and sit-ups in the hotel, carried your own luggage and golf clubs, and used the stairs instead of the elevator.
Cold rainy weather is beginning. Good thing you have that gym

membership and can do the indoor machines when it's too unpleasant outside.

This evening you normally go fly fishing along the stream, but you're tight on time, so you go to the gym for a quick weight-training workout. Not the same as a good long hike fishing, but at least you did your body some good and were able to credit yourself with an exercise day in your diary.

Your true desire was to go on the men's hunting weekend, but you've been gone from the family too much already. Instead you took the family camping. To make it more active, you opted for walk-in tent sites so you and the kids got more exercise hauling gear. You all went exploring the nearby hills for minerals. It was a great weekend – family time, a good amount of physical activity, and an outdoor experience.

Improve your fitness. After a while of performing the same exercise, you become very efficient with the movements, more skilled, better able to do the exercise at a more intense level. Focusing on one activity is important for people who compete in a sport or even recreational exercisers who participate in occasional sport challenges like a long fundraising bicycle ride. In fact, it's good to temporarily drop some activities to prepare for a major sporting event or season. Lots of practice progressively building endurance and intensity with one sport is great for fitness – at least for the physical requirements of that specific type of exercise. On the other hand, too much focus on one activity limits overall fitness.

Adding other forms of exercise is the best way to continue developing your fitness. Each new activity will help you learn a new set of skills, emphasize different muscles, stress your heart and lung function differently, and stimulate brain growth. Fitness spreads. Your body becomes conditioned across body areas and body functions. You reduce or decrease the risk for a greater variety of illnesses or injuries. Becoming more fit sets up a positive spiral: the fitter you are the more willing you'll be to try other physical activities. Fitness is a gateway to an active lifestyle.

Aerobic fitness. Exercise for aerobic fitness is any activity with repeated movements that uses large muscles and requires an increase in oxygen beyond normal. Doing aerobic exercise at least a few times a week will make your heart muscle and the muscles involved in breathing stronger. The flow of blood, nutrients, and oxygen becomes more efficient, allowing more muscular activity and less fatigue. Risk for heart and vascular disease is decreased, high blood sugar is reduced, and weight is reduced. Aerobic exercise also increases strength in muscles, especially those specific to the exercise, although not as much as strength training.

For exercise to produce an aerobic fitness benefit you must increase the demand on your cardio respiratory system. In other words, to exercise your heart and lungs beyond a resting or normal activity level. Overload is the technical term in exercise and sports science for such an increase. That point is usually defined by a specific heart rate. The key to improving aerobic fitness is to cycle between low aerobic work, long endurance episodes, high intensity intervals, and recovery. To measure heart rate and the aerobic cutoffs and for instruction on varying intensity of aerobic exercise, refer back to Chapter 10 on exercise intensity.

The best aerobic activities are ones that suit your skill, fitness, budget and other practical and health considerations. See Figure 12.1 for a variety of aerobic activities listed roughly in order of popularity.

Not surprisingly, walking is the most common form of exercise. Walking can be aerobic. People are designed physically to tolerate long bouts of walking. It's cheap. You can start from your front door. You can use it for transportation. It can be social or solitary. And it requires no equipment or extraordinary skill. Walking is a good beginning for anyone, especially people who are unfit and have not exercised regularly in a long while.

Racquet sports like tennis and racquetball and team sports like basketball, soccer, and volleyball vary body movements, change intensity and create group interaction. More fitness and skill are required for these sports compared to walking, hiking, cycling and aerobic machines. Cross-country skiing and kayaking create upper body fitness. Some people enjoy using special outdoor gear in sports like these. Dancing can be a good total body aerobic workout and a way to combine exercise with a partner or social recreation. More energy can be expended with aerobic dance as skill level increases. Swimming is a great example of an aerobic exercise that is not weight bearing and consequently good for people who are recovering from injury and want to avoid over stressing themselves with too much walking, hiking, running, etc. Some activities such as downhill skiing emphasize muscle strengthening, but also produce short periods of aerobic effort.

Some activities on this list might not seem vigorous enough to be considered aerobic. Others might seem extremely intense. Only a heart rate monitor or other rating system for exercise intensity will verify that a specific activity, performed the way you do it, is indeed good for aerobic fitness.

Aerobic exercise in approximate order of popularity
Walking
Cycling – road bike
Hiking
Fishing – walking stream in waders, walking riverbank or lakeshore
Running, jogging, trail running
Swimming
Indoor aerobic machines: treadmill, elliptical, Nordic track, rowing
Aerobic classes, either live supervised classes or unsupervised classes via exercise TV, videos, or gaming devices (Nintendo Wii). Examples include: step aerobics, Spinning, Jazzercise, Zumba dance, power yoga, kick boxing, walking in place, water aerobics
Golf
Hunting
Dancing
Stair climbing
Mountain bike
Ball sports and team sports: tennis, baseball/softball, basketball, volleyball, racquetball, soccer, badminton, handball, hockey, squash
Skiing, downhill or cross country
Snowboarding
Frisbee
Skating: inline, roller, ice
Kayaking, canoeing, rowing
Snow shoeing
Calisthenics (e.g., jumping jacks)
Jumping rope

Figure 12.1 Many types of physical recreation can create aerobic fitness.

Muscle strength. Exercise for muscle strength is any activity that creates a resistance to contracting muscles usually by lifting, pulling, or pushing weight. Muscle size, strength, and endurance for muscular activity are increased. Tendons and ligaments also gain strength with strength training that bends joints. Stronger supporting tissue around joints protects one from injury. Bones are stressed by muscle strengthening exercise and consequently bone density is increased and the risk of osteoporosis is decreased. Posture and balance are improved especially with leg strengthening exercise. Being stronger helps control back pain, joint pain, and soreness. Stronger muscles help one to function in daily activities and keep one more independent while aging. Simple movements like climbing stairs and rising from a chair are easier. Gardening, housework, travelling, shopping – anything that requires pushing, pulling, carrying will be easier and less tiring.

Any exercise or sport uses muscle strength. To perform better or excel at an activity one needs to increase maximum strength, to increase the ability to exert force quickly – power, and to increase tolerance for repeated muscle contraction – endurance. Competitive athletes need to include strength training in their training regimen. But ordinary recreational athletes and sports participants should include strength training to enhance enjoyment and protect against injury. The skier who does leg strengthening in the gym will ski more vertical feet in a day and be less likely to tweak his or her knees than the skier whose leg strengthening is limited to on-the-hill skiing.

Strength training will encourage weight loss. As muscle size increases, the amount of muscle tissue relative to fat tissue increases. Because muscle burns more calories than fat, the metabolic rate, or amount of caloric energy expended by the body at rest, increases. The act of doing strength training uses some calorie energy, but the effect of larger muscles lasts all day, not just during exercise. Muscle also weighs more than fat and increases in muscle size can be visible. This makes many people worry that exercise will cause a weight gain rather than weight loss. Not to worry. Increasing muscle tissue should be offset by the energy cost of exercise and the loss of fat tissue. In fact, one could say the problem of being overweight is not being "too fat", rather not being "musclely" enough. Although strengthening exercise does not burn as many calories and does not exercise the heart and lungs as much as aerobic exercise, it does help reduce cardiovascular and metabolic disease above and beyond any aerobic exercise you do. Also, strength training changes one's physique and supports aerobic exercise by creating the strength to go harder and longer and feel less tired and sore.

Muscle strengthening can be done in the fitness center with free weights or weight machines. The same equipment, like dumbbells or barbells can be used at home. Low cost strengthening can be done with special rubber bands available at sports shops or with homemade materials such as water jugs filled with water or sand. Exercises such as push-ups, sit-ups, lunges, and squats strengthen large body areas by resisting gravity with body weight. Muscle "toning" classes and videos focus on strengthening without equipment. By not needing gear, these exercises are portable and consequently strength work can be maintained when away from home. Some kind of strengthening is one of the most common forms of exercise.

If you are serious about improving strength, you will need to work out regularly – about three times a week. Strength training twice a week might be enough to maintain increases in strength once you've improved your fitness, but not enough to progress further. It's important to have recovery days in-between strength workouts. Of course, another advantage of frequent strength workouts is they will become a habit. Time wise, a basic strength program should not be a great burden. It can be short, around half an hour.

Flexibility. Flexibility is the freedom to move and to fully stretch at the joints. Poor flexibility is when movement is restricted and inhibited. Stretching exercise improves flexibility and gives your body a better "range of motion". That means more freedom to move your body further and to feel less tight or sore. It's easier to reach, twist, bend, lean, squat, and straighten. On a practical level, ordinary movements are easier when you are flexible: taking things off shelves, bending over to tie your shoes, getting in and out of the car, dressing and undressing. Being flexible does not create aerobic fitness or strength, but it makes it a lot easier and more fun to engage in those types of exercise. More importantly, being flexible helps to prevent injury like muscle strain after a hard aerobic or strength workout. People with flexibility issues who are prone to tight, sore muscles have to skip too many exercise sessions. Being flexible helps you be more consistent with an exercise schedule. Thus, flexibility also is good for making an exercise habit.

Stretching exercises improve flexibility by elongating muscles with slow, deliberate movement held in place while sensing a slight pulling in the muscle. All body areas from head to toes can be stretched: the neck, shoulders, arms, wrists, fingers, chest, trunk, back, legs, knees, ankles and feet. At a minimum, stretch major body areas and muscles specific to your sport or exercise. Stretching can be done formally in a yoga class or informally at home standing and lying and at work sitting in the desk chair. No special gear or skill is needed to practice stretching.

Stretching is a natural activity that people do because it feels good. It's invigorating to stretch. It's not hard work and doesn't have to take much time. Nonetheless, of the three types of fitness – aerobic, strength, and flexibility – stretching is the hardest exercise habit to form. The main problem is simply attitude – people think stretching isn't exercise. Well, it may not burn a lot of calories or take much time, but clearly being flexible is part of physical health and enables other forms of exercise. In fact, stretching does meet the definition of exercise – it's physical activity that is done intentionally for the sake of recreation, pleasure, and fitness.

If it helps you to justify the extra time to stretch, be sure to include good stretching episodes in your exercise diary and count them toward your goal of increasing exercise frequency and time - the two basic parameters of exercise behavior you must increase to form a strong habit.

It will also help to create some cues or a ritual to remind you to stretch regularly. A morning ritual of stretching, stretching before every walk, building a stretch break into your workday – some routine that makes stretching a regular and speaking technically, a high frequency behavior will help make it a habit. If you only stretch in response to infrequent cues like feeling tight or sore, you'll struggle to make it a habit. More importantly, instead of developing true flexibility, you will just be doing damage control from muscle strain. Like other forms of exercise, after some time has passed with regular stretching, you will look forward to it and feel bad when you don't stretch.

Tips On Adding New Types Of Exercise

Make gradual changes. To add a second type of exercise, all you must do is do it on one day next week. Don't worry about how long you do it or how well you do it. Just do enough to justify entering it in your exercise diary. The goal is simply to start practicing the new behavior. Gradually increase the frequency. After doing it once, do it again, then again. Any type of aerobic, strength, or flexibility exercise should be credited on your record, so adding something new doesn't necessarily mean you must increase your total exercise time right now.

Choose an activity to balance your fitness. Ideally you should do a combination of activities that builds strength, aerobic fitness and flexibility. Pick a new type of exercise that adds to your fitness as opposed to something that copies your normal workout. Hiking is a nice nature oriented activity. But if you already have a walking habit, the boost to your fitness by adding hiking will not be as much as if you started a weight training program at the gym. Walking and weight training would be a great combination of two types of fitness training – aerobic and strength.

Another approach would be to add an exercise that emphasizes a different part of your body. The walker who starts kayaking will have two aerobic activities, but in total will enjoy a more full-body workout, as both arms and legs will be exercised. If you enjoy weight training with free weights and add a Pilates class, you would enjoy regular muscle strengthening plus an extra emphasis on center core muscle strength.

Do some exercise in the outdoors. Despite all the advantages of physical recreation in the outdoors, about half of exercisers only exercise indoors. The participation rate outdoors is even lower for women and older adults.

If your regular exercise is indoors, make your second activity something outdoors. Outdoor recreation refers to activities outside of the home and fitness center, in nature or outdoor urban settings. Hiking, hunting, fishing, mountain biking, skiing, snowboarding, trail running and ocean and lake water sports are nature-based activities.

Road biking, walking in town, inline skating, volleyball on the school playground, and backyard swimming are outdoor urban activities. Bird watching, camping, sailing, scuba diving, snorkeling, snowshoeing, waterskiing, backpacking – there are so many options to be physically active outdoors.

People who participate in outdoors recreation exercise longer and more vigorously than indoors and they like exercising more. It's hard to work out on an exercise machine for more than a short time, but a day hike, golf game, or fishing trip can keep you on the move for hours. Outdoor recreation can be a good way to add those important days of endurance exercise. Physical movement outdoors when walking for instance is better for muscle strengthening and joints compared to easy steady footing on a treadmill. More calories are burned outside – a headwind facing a cyclist takes more energy than an indoor exercycle. People tend to vary walking or moving speed outdoors, which burns more calories than a steady speed on an exercise machine.

Doing one activity creates a connection to the outdoors and in turn, a willingness to try other activities. Fishing, camping, running, biking, and hiking in particular are popular "gateway" activities – meaning people who participate in one of these are more likely to engage in other outdoor activities, leading to higher activity levels overall. Over time, outdoor recreation can lead to a lifestyle that is more active. Day trips, vacations, holidays can be designed around the type of physical recreation that is available. Would you vacation to try a new gym? Of course not. But you might make a vacation a river rafting trip or a tour by bicycle.

Besides the fitness benefits, people enjoy the feelings of being physically active outdoors. It's fun. There is a sense of discovery and maybe a physical challenge. It's an escape from normal demands, normal environments. Connecting with nature especially can feel spiritual, mystical. And outdoor recreation can be a good way to connect with family and friends. If you have children, getting outdoors can start them on a path to being physically active as adults.

If you do not have a partner for outdoor activity or you do not know how to get started – two common problems – check your local news sources for nature outings. Most communities have organizations that feature nature walks, wildlife viewing, beginning bike rides, etc. Outing clubs and local chapters of national organizations like the Sierra Club, have activity calendars online where you can sign-up for a group trip or day outing. Many of the large outdoor gear specialty stores offer workshops and instruction for outdoor recreation. There is a learning curve to making the outdoors a bigger part of your life, but help is available.

Join a fitness center. Having said you should add outdoor exercise if you only work out in a fitness center, the reverse strategy can be helpful as well. Most fitness centers offer weights for strength training, aerobic classes and machines, yoga or stretching classes and maybe a pool. In one location, you can try a variety of exercise. If you're not sure what to do, there will be other people to observe and learn from. Fitness centers can be a body image challenge if you think you look bad exercising, look too fat or too out of shape. Check the chapters on Self-Talk and Become Hardy for techniques to handle those feelings.

Combine activities for endurance. Recall that an endurance day once per week is the best first step to create variety in exercise intensity (Chapter 10). If you are struggling to stretch your usual exercise to an endurance session, try combining different activities, one after the other to make the time. A popular mix among my clients was walking or cycling to the fitness center, working out there, and then returning home under their own power. How about a mini-triathlon: swim in your pool, get on the bike for a ride to the local park, and finish with a trail hike. See Chapter 10 for other examples.

Find a "natural" way to exercise. Naturalistic exercise is daily activities of living that enhance physical fitness; exercise with a purpose. Walking to the store, raking leaves, and shoveling snow. These are everyday jobs that have the extra benefit of being good for your body. An aerobics class, golf game, weight training circuit. These are programmed, scheduled activities designed strictly for physical recreation and fitness. Our biological ancestors did not need programmed exercise because all daily necessities were accomplished with manual labor. Now mechanized transportation and labor-saving devices have removed most opportunities to work our bodies the way they were designed. To find a "natural" way to exercise is to pass up a modern convenience and do the chore using your own power. Although it's less time efficient, you are able to squeeze in an extra short bout of physical effort while accomplishing something you need to do anyway.

Walking to work, shop, or to bus and train stops is the simplest form of natural exercise. Whenever possible try walking to your destination instead of driving. Using public transportation is a good way to force yourself to do extra walking. Going by bicycle is another natural mode of travel. Try getting past the practical problems of bicycle commuting, like having the right clothes and cleaning up at work. Clean up your self-talk if you worry about having a professional image as a bicycle commuter. If there isn't a safe and friendly walking route nearby, try parking the car in a location central to your errands or entertainment and walk from place to place. Don't look for the closest parking spot at the shopping mall. Force yourself to walk a bit. The time you lose probably won't be more than the time wasted by circling the parking lot.

Try other short bouts of manual labor. A wearable activity monitor can be a good reminder and incentive to keep moving during the day. Use the stairs instead of the elevator. Carry your groceries to the car. Better yet, carry your groceries home walking with a backpack. Shovel snow rather than use the snow blower. Do the yard work yourself instead of hiring the boy next door. Resist that self-talk that says it would be easier to drive, easier to hire someone. Every little bit of physical effort burns calories and exercises muscles. Naturalistic exercise adds to the fitness being created by your base, more formal exercise program.

Change activity with the seasons. It's hard to keep up bike riding during winter if the temperatures are freezing and the roads icy. Hiking midday in desert regions during summer is too hot. People who face dramatic weather changes with the seasons naturally learn to find alternative activities. Skiing and other winter sports in cold regions, indoor exercise and swimming in hot regions. Fewer hours of daylight during winter also forces people to change their exercise, maybe switching to neighborhood walks after work instead of bicycling on dark roads. It goes without saying that for a strong exercise habit, one cannot surrender physical activity when less friendly seasons arrive. And seasonal change is a good thing. It balances physical fitness, makes you more flexible and adaptable, and is refreshing.

When I moved from New England to Northern California, I was surprised to find that most of my new cycling friends only cycled. If it was a miserable winter day, the bike stayed inside and so did they. Since it would turn sunny and pleasant in a day or so, there was no need to have a back-up exercise plan and consequently, they had no tradition of exercise variety. But even in places like California, there is enough change in weather and daylight to justify participating in other activities. If you live in such an environment, let the new season force you off your usual routine. Don't rigidly stick to a year schedule of the same old thing. Get into something different that suits the weather. Take a break from your normal activity to enjoy something different.

Try an activity that takes skill. How about trying an activity that takes more skill? Walking, hiking, swimming and the treadmill are examples of good fitness activities that do not necessarily require much physical skill. Tennis, skiing, and soccer require more balance, agility, and coordination.

Balance refers to shifting the body in space and regaining position, keeping the body stable and under control while moving. Dancing, catching and throwing balls, ice skating, casting a fishing line, step aerobics, and cross-country skiing are popular activities that require a lot of balance. Balance can be practiced intentionally with exercises of standing on one leg and lifting weights while standing or sitting on balance cushions or balance balls.

Agility refers to rapidly and accurately changing body position. Ball games that involve running in one direction, then turning and running in another require agility.

Coordination uses senses like sight in conjunction with moving. Serving a tennis ball, kicking a football, turning skis to avoid a hazard, dancing, and riding a mountain bike on narrow trails require much coordination.

These physical skills are not directly related to improved cardiovascular or musculoskeletal health as are aerobic fitness, strength, and flexibility exercise. But a new skill is the physical equivalent of doing puzzles or brainteasers. It's a cognitive boost and grows parts of the brain that control motor skills. And of course, higher skilled activities can be great fun, which rewards participating in them.

All these fitness skills can be learned and improved with practice and as result, other sports will be easier and more tempting to try.

Create a good attitude. Having a good attitude and being open to change will make it easier to add variety to your exercise. People who are open to change are prone to feeling bored when doing the same thing over and over. They prefer new experiences and find the newness in and of itself to be exciting and pleasurable. Facing new challenges stimulates feelings of achievement and competence.

In contrast, people who are low on openness prefer consistency and predictability. They feel uneasy and cautious when facing unfamiliar situations. And they might feel anxious and worried about being able to cope. Consequently, people on this end of the continuum tend to avoid being pushed outside of their comfort zone, whereas people on the other end embrace a little discomfort for the sake of excitement and thrill. Where do you fall on this trait?

Clean-up your self-talk. You can create more of an open attitude by using the basic coping strategies presented throughout this book. Starting with self-talk (Chapter 7), what do you say when attempting a new type of activity? Are your thoughts helpful or not helpful? Are you too preoccupied with worrisome thoughts? Are you making up excuses to avoid getting out of your comfort zone? It's normal to worry about injury or being incompetent when trying a new sport.

Try responding with alternative helpful self-statements. Emphasize rational thoughts and personal effectiveness: "I can do this," "With more practice, this will be easier," "It's good for me to try something different," "I'm doing the best I can; it's okay not to be perfect," "Just because I feel scared doesn't mean this is dangerous." Try the reframing technique: for example, interpret sensations like increased heart rate and dread before starting that scary new activity as part excitement rather than all fear; interpret sensations of going fast, as on a bicycle, as being playful rather than being out of control.

Take advantage of social support. Let other people help you learn a new activity, loan you equipment and encourage you to experiment. People are more likely to attempt a scary looking activity if other people are doing it. Being around other people who engage in seemingly challenging sports can make one start thinking of them as normal and doable.

Work on your hardiness. To become more open is like the process of becoming more hardy (Chapter 11). New, challenging sports expose you to adversity. The payoffs for getting outside your comfort zone are the pleasure of the sport and the good feeling of accomplishment for facing the challenge. Going backwards in the chain of events, some of the challenging experiences in the new sport like feeling on the edge of control skiing start to feel fun. In the long run, being more hardy will remove psychological barriers to new recreation and of course, will improve your exercise habit and fitness.

Don't be defensive. Be careful to not reject your options without giving them a chance. It's common for people to rule out a new sport for the reason it looks too hard, too dangerous, too complicated. "No way will I ever try bicycling. I don't want to be hit by a car." "I can't see myself skiing again, I'm just too old." "You won't catch me going to an aerobics class with all those skinny women." This defense mechanism is also known as "self-handicapping." That's the tendency to make something seem harder than it is in order to justify not trying or to complain about a personal weakness to make an excuse in case of failure.

Sarcasm is another form of defensiveness. "My husband wants me to hike up to the hilltop lookout. That's three miles of steep climbing. I say that's why the county park built a road to there." Making light of exercise can be a way to cover-up an underlying fear or feeling of inadequacy. It's better to just admit to your uneasiness and try to deal with it, than to overly limit your exercise options. Something has to give if you are serious about becoming more fit. That might have to be your pride.

Extreme is in the eye of the beholder. The entertainment and advertising media are filled with images of adventurous or "extreme" sports. Think rock climbing, mountaineering, surfing, wakeboarding, horse galloping, white water kayaking, and snowboarding. The defining characteristic of adventure sports is not necessarily the objective difficulty of the sport, it's the feeling involved. The thrill, the courage, and the satisfaction of having tested oneself. Beginner athletes can enjoy the same feelings: skiing a blue intermediate trail could feel as extreme as skiing over a cliff does for another. The common experience is the feeling of thrill.

Be careful to not pooh- pooh thrill seeking: "Those sports are too dangerous. People who do them risk their lives for fun; they're either show-offs or unusually athletic; a normal person could never do that." These are stereotypes, an outside view of adventure sports. The reality is quite different. Most adventure sports participants learned their skills through hard work and a healthy lifestyle – not recklessness. They enjoy the thrill precisely because they avoid unnecessary risks and minimize danger. It's not impossible for a normal person to learn an adventure sport, nor is it radical to seek thrill. Plenty of people, including women and older adults, ski, surf, skate, row, hunt, mountain bike, skin dive, and snowshoe. What is the alternative? To get your thrill from drinking, taking drugs, driving too fast, gambling? Sports are a healthy outlet. Open yourself to the possibilities.

Chapter 13:
Reward Yourself for Exercising

Exercise is intrinsically rewarding, but the built-in rewards might not seem enough to overcome difficulties or to make it feel worthwhile. No wonder lots of people use payoffs or special treats to stay motivated. To be sure, rewards can be an effective to way to encourage a behavior, but that depends on how you reward yourself.

The Nature of Reward

A reward is a consequence, usually pleasurable or desirable, that increases the probability of the preceding behavior. Reward is also called reinforcement, meaning it "reinforces" or strengthens the behavior. If the reward does not motivate the person to repeat the behavior, it's not a reward, even if it seems desirable. So, if you treat yourself to a new pair of walking shoes, but that doesn't make you walk more, the shoes are not a reward. On the other hand, if delaying housework until you walk has the effect of making you exercise more, then housework is a reward, even though it might not seem desirable.

Reward vs. bribe. Reward or reinforcement always follows performance of the behavior. To give yourself something with a promise to do the behavior later is a bribe. A bribe is usually ineffective because the person already has the goodie and there is no loss if the promise is broken. So, to buy some fancy exercise clothes as an inducement to start exercising regularly can be a set-up for failure.

The proper formula is "First I will _____, then I (or someone I designate) will give me or do _____ (this reward). The reward comes after so the person will work for it. Technically, behaviorists say, the reward is "contingent" on the behavior. Administering a reward program is called contingency management. When you administer your own reward program, it takes self-control to withhold the payoff until you reach your goal.

Punishment. Sometimes people punish themselves if they do not exercise, but reward is more effective than punishment. A classic example is the person who joins a gym thinking that he or she surely will use it to avoid being punished by paying a fee for something that is not used. Yet, most gym memberships ARE unused. Because the prospective exerciser has failed once again, he or she accepts the punishment. It's deserved, the person thinks, because after all, this clearly confirms he or she is weak willed, undisciplined or lazy.

Another and more extreme punishment strategy is to forfeit money or belongings, perhaps to a hated organization like the "Society for Everything I Detest". The person is so opposed and repulsed by the organization, surely, he or she would not lose a bet to exercise more.

But even with more extreme consequences, punishment is usually a losing proposition. It makes people feel bad and anxious and consequently interferes with learning. Reward schemes focus on increasing a desirable outcome and are designed to make people feel good. That makes contingency management a positive, hopeful experience.

The theory underlying the effect of reward is proven, but people design poor reinforcement contingencies and blame the theory instead of themselves. Use good reinforcement strategies. So far, I presented three basic points: apply the reward after the occurrence of the behavior, choose a consequence that actually increases the behavior, and focus on reward rather than punishment. Following are some other tips to reward yourself effectively for exercising.

Tips To Use Reward To Your Advantage

Make a commitment. A reward plan is like a contract. Write out your plan rather than just say it silently to yourself. It's too easy to distort or forget promises you make inside your head. Put it on paper or in a note file as an act of commitment and post the contingency plan where you can see it as an exercise cue. Telling other people is a public commitment, which tends to increase the likelihood of follow-through. Send a message to your friends.

Make a specific plan. Make the plan specific and concrete, not vague. "If I set a new record for my longest walk, I will buy myself that new outfit," rather than "If I do well with exercise this week, I will treat myself. "The target behavior to be reinforced should be unambiguous. Being concrete is easy because most exercise behavior is quantifiable and objective, rather than subjective.

Pick an appropriate exercise target. An appropriate target could be one of the basic exercise goals of this program. That includes reaching four days or four hours per week of exercise, and later, six days or six hours. Other basic goals are adding an endurance day, adding a new type of exercise, and practicing high intensity intervals. A reward strategy might help you achieve one of these milestones.

In addition to targeting changes in exercise behavior, you also can target changes in fitness. An example of a fitness goal is a decrease in percent body fat. To achieve that you might put in more hours of endurance exercise plus do strength training with weights. Decreased body fat becomes the endpoint or marker for changes in exercise behaviors that in turn are also reinforced. Weight loss, reaching a higher heart rate zone, and personal record for fastest hike indicate better fitness achieved through behavior change. Rewarding a fitness endpoint can be a very efficient way to reach a variety of antecedent behaviors that create the endpoint.

On the other hand, the behavior to fitness connection is not necessarily reliable. For instance, people can lose or gain weight day to day due to the effects of salt in the food, menstrual cycle, or hydration, rather than how many calories they ate or how much exercise they did. For this reason, to reinforce behavior change is more certain to teach behavior than to reinforce a health outcome. Another issue is how long it will take to be rewarded. Improvements in exercise might have to be sustained for some time before they result in fitness changes. People have immediate and direct control over their behavior, but not necessarily their fitness.

Having said that, most people are looking for a fitness change whether it's losing weight or fitting better in clothes, looking better, lowering blood pressure, or getting off medication. If you want to motivate yourself with a reward, I still recommend you target behavior change – you can get an immediate result. And then if you wish to add another reinforcement contingency, you could experiment with targeting a change in physical fitness as well.

Pick an appropriate reward. A reward is appropriate if you absolutely intend to make it contingent or dependent on following through with your exercise. Don't choose something that you might give yourself anyway. A night on the town might be a good incentive to stick to your exercise plan. But if you don't, will you forfeit that forever? Probably not. So, pick something that you really want, but are prepared to live without until you deserve it. Something that is not a routine or necessary purchase. A good choice might be something special that not only makes you happy, but also encourages even more exercise. Instead of a night on the town, how about a new pair of running shoes. Instead of a concert, how about a computer for your bicycle. Instead of an ice cream sundae, how about a water bottle. Or a heart rate monitor to use on your treadmill instead of a new purse.

A reward does not have to be tangible. It can be an activity or favor from someone else; like your spouse agreed to join you for workouts after you show you're serious about going to the gym. Involving another person can keep you honest and might give you the extra support you need to reach your goal.

Positive and negative reinforcement. Reinforcement does not have to be positive; positive reinforcement is to add something desirable after the behavior. Negative reinforcement, mistakenly thought of as punishment, is a reward, only in the negative – something undesirable is taken away. For instance, you are having trouble getting your workouts. Your husband is willing to take on more house chores when you start adding more days of exercise. For every day you add, he'll do an equivalent extra amount of time in the house. Removing chores is reinforcement in the negative. Other examples of reinforcement in the negative are: removing child care, resigning from committee chores, getting rid of your CPAP machine, stopping medication, giving away old fat clothes. Both positive and negative reinforcement increase the likelihood of behavior.

Exercise purchases should be used as reward. If you are considering a major exercise purchase (gym membership, bicycle, home treadmill, skis, fly fishing pole, kayak) don't buy it until you deserve it. Too many people buy the exercise gear or membership with good intentions to accelerate their exercise habit. These are luxuries; extravagant treats that should come after you've proven you exercise regularly. My recommendation is to not join a gym or buy a big piece of equipment until you hit four days a week of regular exercise. That should include regularly engaging in the sport or activity that you want to support with the purchase. For instance, if you want a fancy treadmill in your apartment, pay for day passes at a gym and use its treadmill long enough to prove a treadmill makes sense for you. Then buy the treadmill. If you're riding an old clunker of a bicycle, stick with it or borrow someone else's bicycle until you prove you will actually cycle regularly. Then buy the new bike. Maybe the old clunker is inefficient and not suitable for long rides. But quality of the workout and pleasure from your equipment are less important than actually engaging in the behavior. To delay a major purchase and use it as a logical consequence for behavior change is good contingency management.

Daily events as rewards. If you have trouble thinking of a good reward or do not like the idea of buying a special treat, try using some daily event as the reward. Recall the technique of "rewarding exercise with lower priorities" in Chapter 6 on prioritizing. That involves delaying a pleasurable daily activity such as taking a shower, opening Facebook or Instagram, or any other high frequency behavior like preparing dinner, until you have exercised. A tension is created so that you want to exercise in order to return to your usual routine. The daily event, even if it is a chore, becomes an immediate reward for making yourself exercise. As explained below, immediate reward is more effective than delayed reward.

Don't delay reward too long. Make a short-term goal and give the reward as soon as possible after the behavior. People are less likely to follow through with longer-term reward schemes. "I will reward myself if I walk six times this week" is more effective than "...if I walk six times a week for the next six months." It's better to buy that new piece of sports equipment right after you make your exercise goal than to wait until next month. Reward yourself for losing five pounds rather than setting too ambitious a weight loss goal. The idea is to break a larger goal into a stepwise plan in order to enjoy quick rewards along the way (see sections on Shaping and Follow a Schedule in Chapter 5).

Longer-term goals can be overwhelming because they are too big. Delayed reward weakens the connection between the behavior and the reward, making the contingency less effective.

Reward yourself more than once. A onetime reward might be appropriate for reaching a milestone. For instance, you might plan something special when the day comes you are able to get off diabetes medication. Or you might celebrate when at last you are exercising six days a week. On the other hand, more frequent reward accelerates the learning of a new behavior. For instance, a positive reinforcement scheduled after each additional day of exercise per week until you reach six days will build up some psychological momentum toward the bigger goal. Breaking down a large goal into small steps allows you to reward progress along the way. Once you reach six days, rewarding yourself the next week for six days, and the next week and the next, in other words repeated reinforcement for the same behavior, will strengthen that behavior more than a onetime reward.

Continuous and intermittent reinforcement. If you have tried to modify behavior in a pet, you might relate to this technique. Let's say you were using a tasty biscuit to train your dog to sit and stay. You probably wouldn't give him a treat just the first time he follows your command. Maybe it was a fluke happening. You would reward him over and over until he understands the connection and learns the behavior. Only then might you space out the reward and give just occasional treats. This technique is a switch from continuous to intermittent reinforcement.

Continuous reinforcement is effective for the initial acquisition of behavior. Switching to intermittent reward helps maintain and strengthen the behavior. How? The person learns to work harder because a larger volume of behavior must occur before the reward is administered. At the same time, the person accommodates to periods without reinforcement and will be less likely to give up when the external, artificial payoffs come to an end.

A classic example of the power of intermittent reinforcement is playing a slot machine. The player learns to continue putting money into the machine, the faster the better, because eventually the machine will pay. If slots were on a continuous reinforcement schedule, such that the player was paid with each pull of the lever, what would happen when the machine stopped paying? The player would stop, of course, because the expectation of being rewarded was no longer fulfilled. An intermittent schedule of reward is more powerful for maintaining the behavior because the person never knows when it will come or knows the behavior must be repeated a lot to earn the reward.

Withdrawing or ending reinforcement altogether is appropriate when you believe the behavior is strong enough to continue without an extra incentive. For instance, when your dog sits on command reliably, you could eliminate the biscuit reward. People tend to error on the over-confident side and end reinforcement prematurely. It can be a nuisance or even a threat to self-pride to depend on a reward. Nonetheless, it's best to continue it for a while to strengthen the behavior.

A good reward plan breaks down a goal into steps, specifies how often the reward will be given and a time to phase out reward. This is called a schedule of reinforcement.

Who should reward you? A reward is effective because it is withheld until the behavior is performed. In theory, it should not matter who delivers the reward, you or another person, so long as it is truly contingent on the behavior. In practice, it is less complicated to administer the reward yourself. The contingency plan will be between just you and your behavior, no public disclosure or dependency on others. The challenge of self-reward is to control yourself, to be honest and to follow through with the contingency. That means not rewarding yourself if you do not deserve it.

Instead of relying on self-control, an alternative is to ask a friend or other support person to be the one to provide the reward. In addition to the incentive of the reward, you will be held accountable to another person, which will prevent you from cheating and will intensify your desire to succeed. Moreover, anyone you pick probably would want you to earn the reward and therefore would encourage you to make your goal. In total, you would receive a double reward: the payoff you arranged plus social reinforcement in the form of praise from your support person.

A simple reward technique would be to deposit something with the other person, to be repaid upon completion of the behavior. That could be money or a personal possession, such as the new MP3 player or your TV that is taking too much time away from exercise. Be careful of this approach, as it resembles punishment. Better would be if your support person is so inclined, and would agree to do you a favor for reaching your goal, such as a night on the town or to take you on the hike you always wanted to do.

Using someone else in a reward scheme is challenging. It involves revealing your struggle and drawing attention to your health or fitness. It creates a dependency and says to the other person, "I need someone else to help control my behavior." Since you've failed before, there is a risk that not only will you be unrewarded, but you will disappoint your support person. It's worth thinking carefully about including a support person. Review the chapter on social support (Chapter 9) for further advice.

Design Your Reward Plan

Examples of exercise reinforcement plans are shown in Figure 13.1. Remember, the target behavior should be specific and objectively measurable. Notice these exercise targets cover basic goals for increasing exercise time as well as variety in exercise type and intensity and improvements in fitness. The types of rewarding consequences include examples of using special treats as well as daily events that are withheld until the exercise behavior is performed. Reinforcement can also be "negative" in the sense of removing something undesirable as shown in Example 6. The reinforcement schedule refers to the frequency and timing of reward. In Example 3, the time frame is unspecified, probably because the exerciser thinks the prospect of hiking with her boyfriend is powerful enough without intermediate rewards to make her increase her walking time. All the other examples use repeated reward with a plan to phase it out when the exerciser demonstrates some consistency. Except in Example 7, the person opted to continue with intermittent reward indefinitely. It might be best to prepare for the possibility of regressing, like Example 2 in which the exerciser must recover his or her fitness before receiving another reward.

It helps to write out a rationale for the reward plan, as shown in the Comment section. If you can't explain the plan in simple words, you probably need to re-work the contingency and reinforcement schedule. Also, having it in writing will help you commit to the plan. Create a form like this for yourself and try rewarding yourself for exercise.

Example reward plans			
Target behavior	**Consequence**	**Reinforcement schedule**	**Comment**
1. Exercise 4 days this week	Download a new app for my phone	A new app each week I make 4 days until I make 4 days, 8 weeks in a row	I spend too much time playing with my phone. I'll use it as an incentive to be more consistent with exercise
2. Lose 10 pounds	Have a session with a personal trainer	Schedule 2 sessions with a trainer each week that I lose 1 lb. or more until I've lost 5 lbs. Then 1 session for each lb. lost until I've lost 10 lbs. If I gain weight, I have to re-lose it before resuming the reinforcement schedule.	I'm seeing a trainer hoping to get motivated, but not following through with her plan. I really like my training sessions, so by reversing the contingency – exercise (and lose weight) first, I can use them as a reward to motivate myself.
3. Build up my endurance for long walks. Do a 2-hour walk.	Hike with my new boyfriend.	Lengthen my endurance day an extra 15 minutes per week until I can walk 2 hours.	My boyfriend loves to hike and I want to enjoy that with him, but I need to get in shape.

Target behavior	Consequence	Reinforcement schedule	Comment
		Then let my boyfriend take me on his favorite hike.	
4. Use my dumbbells and weight machine at home more often: Do a strength workout 3 times per week	Download a video	Each night I've done my workout, download a video; no video on any other day until I have been consistent with the workout for 4 weeks in a row.	I watch a lot of videos that probably take too much time away from being healthier. I'll make videos a reward for sticking to my exercise plan
5. Stretching and physical therapy exercise when I return home from work	Open Facebook	Every day, no Facebook until I have done my exercise. Continue this until my therapist says I'm done	I'm addicted to Facebook and tend to do it before other things I need to do and end up not having enough time to exercise. I'm procrastinating on physical therapy. I need to do to get over my knee injury
6. Six hours of exercise	Quit volunteer jobs	Turn in my resignation after 4 consecutive	It's time to prioritize my health and me,

Target behavior	Consequence	Reinforcement schedule	Comment
	(treasurer for soccer league, school library committee)	weeks of 6 hours exercise	but I'm afraid to give-up other activities until I prove I'm committed to exercise. Dropping some volunteer work will be a relief.
7. Ride my bike 3 times a week	Buy one new cycling garment	At the end of every month with 3 rides each week	I'm riding regularly, but afraid I'll back track.

Figure 13.1 A good reward plan breaks down a goal into steps, specifies how often the reward will be given and a time to phase out reward.

Adjust your plan. If you didn't follow through with your exercise plan, revise your strategy rather than abandon reinforcement altogether. Consider the consequence you chose. Is it a powerful enough incentive? By definition, it may not be a reward if it didn't cause the behavior to be performed. Consider the target behavior or reinforcement schedule. People tend to error on the side of bigger rather than smaller goals. Do you need to break down your goal into smaller steps and focus on a more immediate reward? In the practice of behavior modification as well as ordinary behavior training such as parents learning to manage their children's behavior, some time and testing are required to develop effective reinforcement contingencies.

Switch To Natural Rewards

Physical recreation is a natural activity that is fun and feels good. In time, there are other positive consequences like being healthier, better able to function in daily life, and looking better. But it can take two to four months for exercise to start feeling good, especially for people starting at a sedentary level. Until then, it is perfectly fine and with any luck, helpful to use artificial, contrived rewards to motivate you. External incentives are effective to kick start a behavior, but for something like exercise, the natural rewards should be enough to maintain the behavior after the habit has begun. Use the power of self-talk and thought control to focus on the pleasurable aspects of exercise and the real, intrinsic rewards. Soon you won't have to bother creating extra reward contingencies. Exercise behavior and positive feelings will be automatic.

Chapter 14:
Believe in Your Health

You probably would exercise if you thought your life depended on it. The reality is, your life does depend on exercise. Nearly every chronic illness or disability is caused or worsened by lack of exercise – and nearly every health problem is prevented or improved by exercising more. Although most people already know this, knowing exercise is good for health is not enough for people to change their behavior. But truly <u>believing</u> exercise is important for you personally can be. Instead of waiting for a major illness or disability to give you a wake-up call to start believing, how about becoming a believer now. This chapter will help motivate you to exercise by focusing more on helpful health beliefs.

What Are Health Beliefs?

Exercise is considered a health behavior because its presence or absence predicts health outcomes, such as the occurrence of disease, the risk for death or incapacity for daily function. Health knowledge is information or facts about health and health behavior. Nowadays, people are bombarded with health information. Almost everyone has read or heard that it's healthy to exercise, but only a minority of people exercise enough – this proves that awareness or knowledge clearly is not a good predictor of the behavior. Ironically, as people age they exercise less, even though awareness of health issues increases with age.

Health belief is an opinion about health information. Although most people are aware of health facts, not everyone forms an opinion about the validity or the personal relevance of those facts. But those who do are surer about what causes illness, what its effect will be, or how it should be treated. People make choices based on their beliefs. If you have faith that exercise will make an important difference for you, you will be more likely to choose an active lifestyle.

Why don't people believe more in the health benefits of exercise? The main reason is the benefits don't occur right away and the time separation between exercise and better health makes it hard for the exerciser to connect the two. It could take months for exercise to eliminate the need for medication. The prevention of disease such as heart attack is even more remote time-wise. Not surprisingly, people believe more strongly in the shorter-term benefits of exercise: positive self-esteem, better physical appearance, and weight loss. These are the main reasons people start to exercise. Better health might be on the list of reasons, but not necessarily at the top.

Another explanation is that to <u>not</u> believe bad things might happen if you don't exercise is a psychological coping mechanism. It's called denial; an unrealistic refusal to acknowledge the facts. A health scare is just that, scary, and full of stresses including having to do something you don't want to – exercise. To convince yourself that exercise isn't that important or doable is a way to avoid the situation. Denial saves pride and buys some time to let reality sink in, time to figure out how to change health behavior. But continual denial is not adaptive: the problem worsens as one pretends it does not exist. Minimization, the opposite of exaggeration, is a related coping mechanism – the facts are not denied but the importance of them is downplayed. So, for instance, the reluctant exerciser might believe exercise will help prevent diabetes, but still thinks having diabetes is not that bad.

What Are Your Health Beliefs?

Health experts have identified the types of beliefs that best predict health behavior. Before I present them and give you some tips on how to make your thinking about exercise more health oriented, let's begin by looking at your beliefs at the present time. To that end, I could create a questionnaire with a list of beliefs for you to rate. It might seem strange to say so, but people don't always know what they believe. Beliefs develop over time subconsciously based on experience and evidence to support them.

Remember from Chapter 7 that self-talk is the conscious and concrete expression of underlying mental processes. So, instead of filling out a questionnaire, I suggest simply writing a reply to the following exercise on "Self-Talk About My Health" (Figure 14.1). Do not read the following section that categorizes types of beliefs before answering the questions. Later it will be useful to see which types already appear in your self-talk and which do not. The two questions ask for thoughts that encourage and discourage exercise. Health beliefs can be negative, so it is important to identify typical thoughts that are unhelpful too. Don't think about it too much. Write the answers that come to mind immediately.

Self-Talk About My Health

1. What do I say to myself about my health or risk of illness or injury that motivates me to exercise? For example, "If I don't keep up my walking, I'll have to take more medication."

2. What do I say to myself about my health that makes me skip exercise? For example, "I've been walking for a couple months and my blood pressure is still high. Why bother doing this."

Figure 14.1 Write self-talk that expresses beliefs about exercise and your health

Types Of Health Beliefs

Health beliefs can be categorized into opinions about the personal relevance and threat of health problems, the cost versus benefit of health behavior, and the recommendations for health behavior from other people. All these come together and lead to the belief closest to the actual performance of the behavior – the intention to engage or not engage in that behavior.

Beliefs about susceptibility. People form beliefs about how susceptible they are to disease, disability, or death. If one thinks it's very unlikely they could develop a particular disease, they are unlikely to engage in behavior to protect themselves from that risk. People don't want to feel vulnerable to bad things, so to deny the possibility of poor health and aging can be comforting, though maladaptive. To believe in your own susceptibility, on the other hand, is an act of humility – to admit you are not immune from trouble, that you could develop an illness. If you truly think, "bad things could happen if I don't do something", you're more likely to take action. Feeling vulnerable is okay. The more likely you think you could get sick, the better – at least when there are other constructive beliefs along with it, such as believing that you can take control of your health.

Do you think you could develop a health problem? What has your doctor told you? What troubles are you already facing? Be honest. Did you write any statement in the exercise, "Self-Talk About My Health", that reflects a belief in susceptibility to ill health? Eventually, everyone faces disease and disability. What might worry you? Can you relate to any of these examples?

Examples of Beliefs in Susceptibility
1. "If I stay like this, I could develop diabetes."
2. "If I don't get serious about exercise, my osteoporosis will worsen."
3. "People like me have had strokes. There's no reason it can't happen to me."
4. "I already feel older, I could start slowing down even more if I don't do something about it."
5. "Both my grandfathers had heart disease, so I could too."
6. "I gained weight. At this rate, I'll be obese by the time I'm fifty."
7. "My skin is getting saggy. Pretty soon I'll look like my mother."
8. "My knees are bothering me. I hope I will not need a knee replacement."
9. "I'm having trouble keeping up with the yard work. I seem to be feeling weaker and less energetic."
10. "With my family history, if I don't exercise, I could end up having to take high cholesterol medication too."

Beliefs about seriousness. Is the health problem to which you are susceptible, serious or not serious? Is it life threatening? Would it be terrible or painful if you became ill? How disabled could you become? How much a burden might you be? What do you believe are the consequences of your health issues? Did you identify any consequences in your self-talk about health?

Beliefs about seriousness are the flip side to beliefs about susceptibility. Perhaps you have been told that you are at risk for diabetes, but you may or may not think diabetes is a serious, potentially debilitating condition. Beliefs about consequences are more accurate when one actually faces them. Until then, it's normal for people to downplay or deny negative consequences in order to manage stress. On the other hand, to believe one's life would be seriously, negatively impacted by a health problem should motivate one to do something about it.

Examples of Beliefs in Seriousness
1. "I could go blind or die young from diabetes, like my mother."
2. "If I keep gaining weight, I'll feel a lot worse than I do already."
3. "My bad knees will make me useless around the house."
4. "I'm afraid that if I had a stroke, I'd be a terrible burden to my wife."
5. "When I feel ill, I feel depressed, like I'm not worth anything."
6. "Heart disease is a killer."
7. "I can't fool myself - there is no cure for dementia."
8. "Being lazy will make me a cripple."
9. "If I don't keep up my youthfulness, I won't be able to do the travelling I want."
10. "I'm so proud of myself. Exercising more is keeping me from depending on my children to take care of me."

Beliefs about benefits. The likelihood of taking action to prevent a health problem depends in part on how beneficial the treatment or behavior change seems it will be. If you are convinced that exercising more will improve your health and prevent some dreaded condition, you're more likely to change. On the other hand, if you're fatalistic and think you have no control over your health, then you won't see any reason to try doing something about it. If you think all treatment has to come from the pill bottle, you're not likely to have much faith in behavior change. Do you have positive expectations for the benefits of exercise? Check your self-talk about health.

Examples of Beliefs in Benefits
1. "Being physically active will keep my mind sharp."
2. "The more physically fit I am, the more I can do around the house without depending on others."
3. "Aerobic exercise will help me prevent a heart attack."
4. "Exercising a lot will help me lose weight."
5. "I can get plastic surgery or I can exercise to look better."
6. "All I have to do is walk 30 minutes a day to make a big difference in my blood sugar."
7. "A little bit of inconvenience to exercise is better than a lot of inconvenience from being disabled."
8. "Not only will I look and feel better physically, but exercise will make me feel better about myself as a person."
9. "I can get off medication if I keep up my exercise."
10. "My back pain will improve and hopefully I will avoid surgery if I ride my bike regularly."

Beliefs about barriers. If all the consequences of health behavior were positive, people would not resist change as much as they do. But behavior change can be difficult, so it is important to look at your ideas about what could stop you from exercising. Potential barriers could include the physical effects of exercise, the social or practical aspects of exercise, and personal coping skills or self-confidence. To have some barriers is normal. How much difficulty is too much depends on your other health beliefs. Significant benefits that you may expect from exercise can offset its inconvenience. Mentally, we evaluate behavior change by calculating this cost-benefit ratio.

Motivation to change is greater when the benefits win. How do these two types of beliefs compare in your self-talk?

Examples of Beliefs in Barriers
1. "Putting this much time into exercise will take away from work."
2. "All this record keeping on exercise is a nuisance."
3. "I hate to sweat. How will I cope in front of an exercise class?"
4. "This gym membership will cost me more than I want to spend."
5. "How am I going to walk every day if it rains?"
6. "My husband will have to rearrange his schedule so I can work out. He's not going to like that."
7. "I'm not very coordinated and I'm sure my friends will laugh when they see me ski again."
8. "I'd like to start exercising again, but if I quit like before, I'll end up feeling worse about myself."
9. "It's time to focus on me. I feel pretty confident I can do it."
10. "I've been successful before; I can do it again."

Beliefs of what others think. These are beliefs about what other people think is desirable and what you should do. The other people could be close friends or family, authority figures or celebrities, or some group of people in general. They don't have to give you advice directly in words; they can model what presumably is desirable behavior in their actions. Either way, one forms a belief about what other people think. Such beliefs can motivate behavior change through reward mechanisms. One is social approval for following the person's advice. The other is a feeling of comfort and security by conforming to normal behavior. In simple terms, this process is peer pressure.

Often people are more likely to give in to what others think is desirable than to follow their own reasoning about the costs and benefits of the behavior. Adolescent health behavior is a classic example. In this age range, doing what other kids do is more relevant than doing what is best for health. Cigarette smoking, safe sex, and drinking alcohol, for example, are highly influenced by peer pressure.

In the case of exercise, my experience has been that social group has a huge effect on the likelihood of succeeding. Unfortunately, only a minority of people exercises enough. The chances are that people in your environment will not model the right behavior and may even give negative messages about exercise. Thus, it's important to focus on social approval and positive role models in order to encourage exercise and to offset, what regrettably has become the norm in our society – to act like a sedentary lifestyle is okay.

Did opinions or wishes of others appear in your health beliefs about exercise? Were they for or against the behavior changes you are trying to make?

Examples of Beliefs of What Others Think
1. "Walking is normal. I see a lot of other people walking in the morning."
2. "My friends who are fit take an exercise break every day."
3. "My faith says taking care of my health is important."
4. "I know the neighbors would like me to join them for the walking group."
5. "Dr. Wright has been telling me I need to exercise more."
6. "Other people who are super busy find time to exercise. Even our President exercises."

7. "I see people at the gym who don't seem to care how sweaty they look; they just like working out."

8. "My family thinks I spend too much time puttering around the house instead of being outdoors with them."

9. "My children want me to be more active with them."

10. "Everything I read about health is telling me to get off my butt."

Motivation to comply with others. There is a constant barrage of health advice in our society. Whether you follow it depends on your attitude toward the source of the message. If you care about the person, if you admire the expert or celebrity, if you want approval from someone else, you are more likely to comply with his or her advice. The choice might be easy when your family, doctor, and friends all are telling you to exercise more. But the choice is harder when experts tell you to exercise, but your spouse says, "Don't". Furthermore, people can resist outside pressure to change, even if it's good for them if somehow compliance is a threat to self-esteem or need for independence. The ideal formula for pro-health behavior change is: "Other people think I should exercise and I want to do what they think is best."

Does your self-talk include any thoughts about wanting to do what other people say about physical fitness or about wanting people to approve of the changes you are making?

Examples of Motivation to Comply

1. "My doctor will be really impressed by my exercise next time I see her."

2. "I want to make my children proud of me."

3. "If I get off my butt, maybe my husband will stop pestering me to

use my bike again."

4. "I'm getting a lot of positive feedback for my hard work. That helps me to keep going with my exercise."

5. "People have been encouraging me to not give up on exercise. I want to show them I can do it."

6. "People in the gym know what they're doing. I want to fit in with the crowd and look competent."

7. "I wonder what my trainer thinks. I'm going to work out in-between our sessions so she knows I'm serious about following her program."

8. "My hiking friends will be disappointed if I don't show up for Sunday's hike. I can't let them down."

9. "I have to keep losing this weight. My wife is concerned about my health and she has a right to be. I want to become healthier for myself but also for her sake."

10. "Seems like the best way to meet people here is to get into some sport. I guess it's time to find my old tennis racquet and start playing again. Maybe that way I'll make some friends."

Positive And Negative Health Believer, Which Are You?

By positive or negative I am referring to the helpfulness of health beliefs. Most of the examples above are "positive", meaning they should encourage you to engage in desirable health behavior. The tone of positive health beliefs need not be upbeat or happy. For instance, it would be on the morbid side to think, "I might die if I don't change." But that would be a positive, useful admission for the person who needs to take control of his or her health.

Negative health beliefs can be upbeat on the surface, but negative in the sense of discouraging healthy behavior. To think you'll never get sick might make you feel less anxious, but will not encourage you to change your behavior.

Each type of health belief discussed so far is able by itself to predict health behavior. An even more powerful predictor of health behavior is the combination of different beliefs. When beliefs about illness susceptibility, seriousness, and the benefit or desirability of behavior change all go in the same direction, positive or negative, the likelihood of actually changing behavior is much greater. Conflicting beliefs can sabotage behavior change. For instance, you might think exercise would improve your health, but worry that other people would disapprove of you becoming a fitness enthusiast. As it turns out, most people who think adaptively in one way think adaptively in the other ways as well. Different types of beliefs tend to correlate with each other. Here are a couple examples of putting all the beliefs together in the right direction and wrong direction.

Positive health believer. "I'm really worried that my joint pain will worsen and I won't be able to do things around the house. That would make me more dependent on my husband, more of a burden than I am already. I couldn't stand being disabled. I know I'd have problems with depression again. My doctor says doing muscle strengthening exercise will make a difference – it's not too late to improve my condition. I believe him, because I've seen my friend get over her knee problems without surgery, just by exercising. I dread going to that exercise room in the senior center, but if that's what it takes, I will do it. People around me would be very proud if I do this."

Here is another example that combines all the types of beliefs into a positive attitude toward exercise. "I'm really not in the mood to go out in this weather to ride my bike. But if I skip days like this, it will be all that much harder the next time I'm facing bad weather. Then the whole vicious cycle toward giving up exercise could happen again: bad weather, losing fitness, skipping more exercise. I feel very hardy if I ride in this weather. Besides, the guys think I'm riding today; I'm not going to look like a quitter by not showing up."

Negative health believer. "My doctor has been trying to get me to exercise more. He's using scare tactics by telling me I could have a heart attack if I don't. Maybe it's his obligation to warn patients, but I think he's going overboard. All I have is a little high blood pressure. It's being taken care of by medication. I don't feel sick at all. Anyway, with all the medical problems I had, I've never had a problem getting back to normal. I just don't have the time now to exercise more. If something bad happens to me, it's meant to be; nothing I can do about it."

The negative health believer is doubtful, uses denial and minimization, surrenders control to fate, and consequently is unmotivated to change. These are health beliefs for the ostrich.

How To Modify Your Health Beliefs

Health beliefs are developed over time as a result of experience, accumulation of knowledge and exposure to other people's opinions. Eventually the regular exerciser more strongly believes exercise is important as they learn it reduces ill health. But with the power of self-talk, people can consciously create new health beliefs, correct old ones, and bring them into awareness right away. Self-talk about health can have an immediate and motivating effect on behavior.

Create positive health self-talk. Now that you are familiar with the types of beliefs that have an important effect on behavior, you can start creating your own. Use the worksheet (Figure 14.2) to write some helpful and reasonably believable statements in each category. Here are some tips on formulating statements.

Susceptibility. This belief is about the relevance of health issues. You have to think you are susceptible to a health problem. If it's difficult to imagine the possibility of an illness, think about being susceptible to other problems with "wellness". For instance, are you worried about becoming less fit, gaining weight, not being as productive or strong, aging prematurely, having to give up sports, etc.

Severity. Don't minimize the severity of health problems. Thinking you might die is morbid, but there is nothing wrong with a little catastrophizing so long as you balance it out with the benefits of behavior change.

Benefits. Eliminating hypertension, obesity, or high blood sugar would be a major positive outcome for behavior change. But these benefits can take a while to reach. In the meantime, becoming more healthy and fit leads to many short-term consequences. Among these are psychological benefits such as more positive self-esteem, more positive body image, better mood, less stress, more mental alertness. To form expectations for short-term outcomes like these increases motivation.

Barriers. Barriers are predictions about the difficulty or negative consequences of behavior change. Adaptive health beliefs are not supposed to be rosy and unrealistic. You should acknowledge the barriers rather than pretend they don't exist. If you expect difficulty, the difficulty will not be as bad when it comes. Unexpected difficulty can make it harder to change. It's okay to balance barriers with positive expectations for personal effectiveness. For instance, "It will be really hard to find time in the evening to exercise, but I can do it."

What others think and motivation to comply. Normalize positive health behavior by looking for it in others. Notice people walking, riding on the bike path, and going to the fitness center. Tell yourself that it's normal to exercise. Don't put down people who exercise or tell you to exercise. Instead of being defensive, try the opposite attitude. Tell yourself you want to be like those exercisers, that you want to please people who care about your health. Thinking that you care what others do or want you to do, points you in that direction.

Create positive health beliefs in all the categories. If you already have one motivating belief, you are off to a great start. But it's the combination of different types of beliefs that best predicts health behavior. Rehearse your statements and practice them at key moments when you might otherwise skip an exercise episode. Use positive health beliefs to combat resistance to exercise. After all, the most important reason to become a regular exerciser is to have a healthy body. Say your health beliefs with feeling even if they seem awkward at first. Re-read Chapter 7 for other tips on making your self-talk more helpful.

You're more likely to believe something if you have information to back it up. So, read literature on exercise and health. Popular press reports on health issues almost always cite exercise as a factor for disease prevention. Include that information in your self-talk. Do some research on how exercise might help you improve your health issue. Add that to your self-talk about benefits.

My Positive Health Beliefs	
Susceptibility	
Severity	
Benefits	
Barriers	
What others think	
Motivation to comply	

Figure 14.2 Use this worksheet to write positive self-talk about exercise and your health.

Chapter 15:
Don't Give-Up Your Exercise Habit

Learning to exercise is hard and unfortunately, learning to quit is easy. First one minor slip, then another, then the dread of having to start again, then discouragement, and finally - letting go of exercise completely. Complex health behaviors like exercise rarely are maintained non-stop without interruption. The challenge is to control interruptions and recover quickly back to regular exercise instead of spiraling into a total relapse. This chapter is designed to help you anticipate threats to your exercise and to be prepared with the resolve needed to overcome them. As worrisome as slips from exercise may be, you will learn that the art of recovering from slips is itself learned behavior. Consequently, slipping and practicing recovering is a necessary, even desirable requirement to deepen your habit.

How Many People Give-up Exercise?

Most people have friends or family who have lost a lot of weight, only to regain it or who have quit smoking only to start smoking again. It turns out that to maintain regular exercise in the long term is about as difficult and unlikely as to maintain other improvements in health behavior. Giving up exercise is a familiar story. Indeed, some people don't even try to exercise because they've given up so many times before that they do not want to feel like a failure again.

Some time ago health researchers began to compile data on the number of people who started using addictive substances again after having successfully quit through a medical or behavioral treatment program. It turns out that most people start abusing drugs and alcohol not long after treatment ends even though supposedly they are cured.

The probability of regressing is basically the same for all types of drug abuse. Smokers relapse as much as alcoholics and alcoholics relapse as much as heroin users. Commonsense is that hard drugs like heroin should be harder to quit because supposedly they are so terribly addicting. But this turns out to not be the case. Studies of long-term weight loss have shown a similar trend. In the months following successful dieting, many people start regaining weight and later only a small portion have maintained their weight loss. Again, the story for long-term exercise is the same. Within the first few months after achieving regular exercise many people deteriorate to sporadic exercise or completely quit. By the end of the year, only a minority is still exercising regularly. Think of that; it's as hard to keep exercising, as it is to kick a heroin habit.

The relapse curve. To relapse means to give up the new good health behavior, to fall back to the old health risk behavior, and to regress to poorer physical health. The relapse rate from different health behaviors is shown by the graph in Figure 15.1. This is an illustration of the probability of relapse based on a compilation of statistics from clinical studies of weight loss, smoking cessation, alcohol and narcotic addiction, and exercise. It's an illustration of the average trend across behaviors – not meant to be statistically exact – and is called the relapse curve.

The curve begins on the left side at time zero with the 100% of individuals who succeeded at the end of treatment (or self-treatment), meaning all the people who were "cured", improved, or adhering to the new health habit. For substance users, that would include all the people who stopped smoking, drinking alcohol or using heroin or other addictive drugs. For weight loss, it would be people who lost a significant amount of weight. For exercise, it would be people who were exercising most days of the week. Following the curve to the right where the percent of people who maintained health is shown across time reveals the relapse effect. That would include people who were continuously abstinent from drugs, kept off a significant portion of their weight loss, and still regularly exercised.

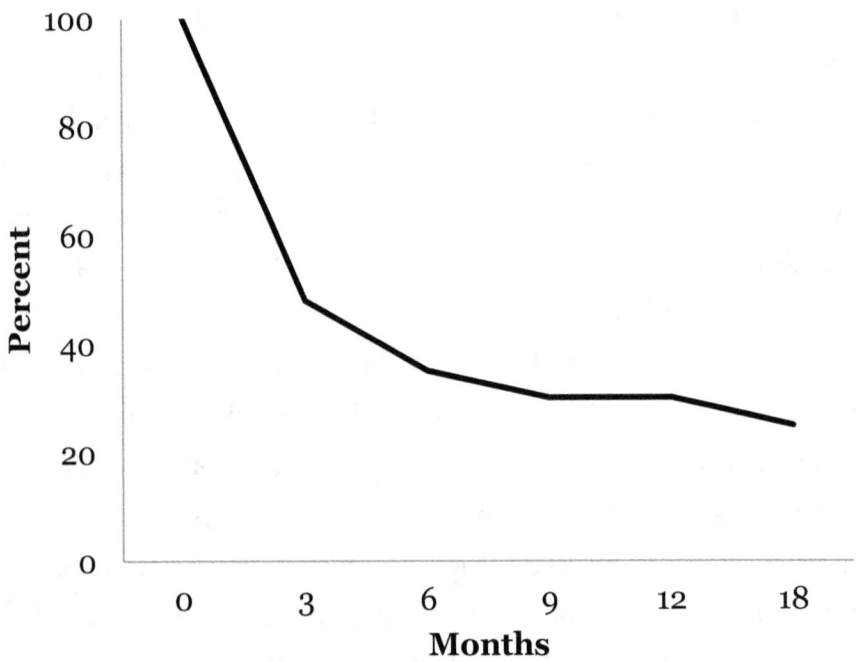

Figure 15.1 The Relapse Curve shows the percent of people who maintained their behavior change during the months after their initial success (starts with 100% of the successful people at Month zero).

What does the relapse curve teach us?

Maintenance is different than treatment. Behavioral interventions to change health habits can be divided into a "treatment" phase and a "maintenance" phase. Treatment is the education phase when you are receiving help from a personal trainer, weight control program, exercise buddy or this book to establish new exercise behavior patterns. The relapse curve in Figure 15.1 begins at time zero after succeeding, when supposedly you are ready to continue "on your own" and to keep what you achieved. This is the maintenance phase.

In the early days of drug rehab and weight loss programs, it was naively assumed that after intensive professional help, people would stay cured. The stark contrast between treatment success followed by relapse emphasizes that to maintain behavior change requires different skills and coping techniques than to acquire new behavior. If your progress in this program is similar to most people, you should consistently exercise at a high frequency sometime between three and four months. It is around that time that you will transition to the maintenance phase when you will need to practice coping with slips in your exercise routine.

Maintenance of health behavior change is a basic problem. The exact success rate can vary, but the timeline or trajectory of the drop-off in success is similar across behaviors. No matter how difficult it might be to quit hard drugs versus to quit being sedentary, the odds for staying quit are about the same. This points to a universal problem for the creation of long-term health habits. There isn't something magically evil about exercise specifically. Something bigger than the hassle of exercise is at fault. All these problems of substance use, overweight, and sedentary behavior are fueled by a complex mix of behavioral and biological factors with powerful environmental and cultural pressures to engage in unhealthy behavior. Two implications for you at this time are: One, to maintain your exercise habit requires that you take the challenge seriously and practice the self-management strategies presented below. Two, interruptions to exercise happen. It's normal to feel like giving up. These occurrences do not prove exercise is hopeless or that you have a character defect.

The risk for relapse changes over time. Too many people relapse very quickly after treatment ends. After graduating cured from a residential treatment program and supervision ends, drug and alcohol addicts often relapse soon after going back to the streets where the problem started. After graduating from supervision by a demanding personal trainer, many people have trouble returning to the gym regularly without having to be accountable to someone. People quit positive health behavior anytime but the biggest drop-off is within the first few months after a structured program, regardless of whether it's supervised or not. Figure 15.1 shows that the relapse rate is greatest early during the maintenance phase.

On the other hand, the encouraging finding is that after most of the "failures" have relapsed the drop off flattens around six months. See the right side of the relapse curve. By then just a smaller portion of people are still maintaining the behavior, but the chances any of them will give up during the rest of the year or longer is pretty low. For that reason, if you are serious about making exercise a lasting habit, you must make it past the maximum risk period at the beginning and keep going, month after month. The longer you go, the less likely you will relapse.

It might seem simplistic to recommend that you prevent backsliding by not backsliding. But as a matter of fact, the secret for long-term success boils down to practicing the new behavior longer and longer. In addition to the importance of frequency of practice, considering these data on relapse, we can add that habit strength is also a function of length of practice over time. One wonders if there are special skills or characteristics of the people who make it to the right side of the relapse curve. The strategies of successful maintainers will be presented below.

Type of treatment is not crucial. Some treatment programs and behavior change strategies work better than others resulting in some differences in the exact percent of people who maintain their improvement. Nonetheless, the relapse curve is essentially the same shape across treatments with most people backsliding early on and a smaller group of long-term successes. Applying this to exercise, it could be said that the way you start an exercise habit is less important than how you cope with temptations to give-up. This is good news for people who feel lost over choosing the type of exercise to do – should I join a gym or should I do it on my own, should I use a treadmill or should I do an aerobics class? Yes, it's best to find an exercise that you enjoy or one that will inspire you. It's best to include outdoor activity. It's best to add variety to exercise. But what matters most is how long you keep going.

Why Do People Relapse?

Why would you give up exercise after all the hard work and positive changes to health and self-esteem? It's bewildering. It's irrational and self-defeating to let go of such a positive habit and every time it's happened, you probably felt confused. Unfortunately, most of our explanations err on the side of being overly self-critical. Surely you would have stuck with it if you had good sense and fortitude. The fact you didn't must prove you lack will power, you're weak. If giving up exercise is a resignation to ill heath, then maybe you also are masochistic or even suicidal. This might sound like psychological exaggeration, but irrational behavior can make one turn inward in a very unforgiving manner.

Self-criticism is normal, but it does little good to beat yourself up and fault your personality if you quit exercise. In this section, we will see that new habits are vulnerable to reversals. It is a result of basic processes in learning that affect us all. Simply put, old behavior is never completely forgotten and will return under the right conditions.

The mechanisms underlying relapse in exercise. First, I will briefly summarize the ways in which behavior is changed and then the ways in which old behavior can reappear. The old behavior in the background waiting to reassert itself is sedentary behavior (using the term "sedentary" here, I am including physical inactivity generally). Both behaviors, exercise and the alternative incompatible behavior – sedentary behavior, will be addressed in these examples of learning processes. It's not important to remember the technical terms, but to have a basic appreciation for the forces at work when it comes to relapse.

Learning to change behavior. An undesirable behavior, in this case sedentary behavior, is eliminated and replaced in specific situations with a new more desirable and incompatible behavior, exercise, as a result of "extinction" and "counterconditioning".

Extinction. Let's say 6 o'clock after a hard day of work is one of your typical sedentary times. It's when you rest on the couch reading the news until dinner. After that, you have little motivation to exercise because it's dark and you feel full after eating. The time of day, sight of the couch and feelings of fatigue are cues that habitually trigger your sedentary behavior. Starting now you stop the couch ritual after work. Pretty soon, evening time and the couch no longer compel you to be lazy. Laziness has been put on "extinction;" you have "extinguished" your pre-dinner sedentary ritual.

To use a food example: You have a habit of eating potato chips in the kitchen when you see the bag on the counter. Although your family still keeps chips in the house, you stopped eating them. After a while, you do not have a strong craving to eat chips when you see the bag on the kitchen counter. Extinction is the elimination of a behavior in the presence of a cue that normally triggers that behavior by repeatedly practicing not engaging in the behavior when exposed to the cue.

Counterconditioning. Let's say that one day after returning from work you pass the couch to dress yourself in a walking outfit and head out the door for a walk. You repeat that day after day. After a while you expect a walk before dinner and the sight of the couch or feeling fatigued after work do not stimulate laziness; instead it reminds you that it is time for a walk. You have counterconditioned the cues of the couch and evening time by associating them with a new behavior, an evening walk.

To use the food example: You have a habit of eating potato chips in the kitchen when you see the bag on the counter. You start snacking on carrots and green peppers instead. After a while, you have cravings to snack on raw vegetables in the kitchen, instead of chips. Counterconditioning is when a cue that was associated with one behavior is later associated with another as a result of repeatedly practicing the new behavior in the presence of that cue.

Lapses in behavior change. The undesirable behavior, being sedentary, returns in place of the new behavior, exercise, as a result of "renewal", "reinstatement", or "spontaneous recovery". Other psychological mechanisms can trigger a relapse as well.

Renewal. Let's say you have given up couch lazing at home in favor of taking an evening exercise walk. A time comes when you are working out of town. When you return to your hotel room at 6:00 you see the couch and instead of going for your walk, you vege out with the newspaper. You learned a walking routine at home, but you did not learn it in other situations where you also were accustomed to being a couch potato, like hotels. Consequently, your evening laziness was "renewed" upon exposure to this different context.

With the food example: You have a habit of eating chips at parties and at home. You stop eating chips at home, even though you still see them around the house. Sometime later, you see chips at a party and have a slip on chips. Renewal can happen when a behavior (sedentary behavior) occurs in more than one context, but changing that behavior only takes place in one context.

Reinstatement. Let's say you replaced your habit of couch sitting before dinner with exercise walks. The weather is so horrendous for a couple days, you're forced to stay in and hang out at your former rest stop – the couch. After good weather returned, seeing the couch triggered an expectation to relax and enticed you to skip your walk. Soon you were back to being inactive in the evening. You "reinstated" sedentary behavior by practicing it again, albeit for just a couple times, in the presence of the cues (couch and time of day) that were originally associated with that behavior.

A food example would be: You had a habit of eating chips at parties, but stopped. One weekend camping, a friend persuades you to eat chips and you remembered how great chips taste. The next time you attend a party, you have a strong craving and start eating chips again.

Spontaneous recovery. Let's say that you were consistent for months with taking an evening walk instead of being lazy on the couch. One day for no apparent reason, you skip the walk and vege out for the evening. Again, it happens and soon you are back to not being active after work. This is a "spontaneous recovery" of the sedentary behavior that formerly was associated with cues at home. The old behavior returned after a long while of not performing it. It is assumed that the passage of time is like a new context and the elimination of the original behavior does not generalize or continue to that new context, the later period of time. Similarly, the recently conditioned behavior, evening exercise behavior, does not generalize to the new time context.

A food example is: You were consistent in not eating chips for months. Then one day for no apparent reason, you had a strong craving and ate some. It's assumed that some changes internal or external occurred out of awareness in the new time context that triggered the old behavior.

Lapses in exercise can occur because the association between certain cues in the environment that normally trigger exercise (or not being sedentary) has broken down. Renewal, reinstatement and spontaneous recovery describe how this happens. Remembering these terms is unimportant compared to appreciating the fact that under the right circumstances, it's easy to regress to old behavior.

Reward and punishment. We can also understand slips and relapse from a reward and punishment perspective. What if the rewards that helped to maintain exercise are withdrawn, such as when a supportive exercise partner is no longer available? If the person has no other positive feelings about exercise to rely on, it could slip away. Then the alternatives – being sedentary, less pressed for time, more relaxed – might feel like a relief. Sometimes it just feels good to not exercise. Now reward for exercise has been withdrawn and reward for sedentary behavior has been restored. Remember we are programmed to conserve energy and to be sedentary. It's human nature.

As much as you might want to end the lapse, after slipping into being a couch potato, exercise can feel bad all over again when you restart. Feeling out of shape again, having to give up the pleasure of laziness – these are exercise punishers.

Mental attitude. It's normal and adaptive to regret slipping on exercise, but to exaggerate feelings of regret can trigger a quick spiral into a relapse. Informally you could call this the "I blew it" reaction whereby one unnecessarily takes a minor slip as proof that exercise is hopeless.

A term used in the field of substance abuse is the "Abstinence Violation Effect". A smoker, for instance, who quit for months gave in to temptation ("violated" abstinence") and had a cigarette. Although the smoker feels guilty, the paradoxical "effect" is he or she suddenly gives up trying to resist temptation and starts smoking all over again.

The psychological explanations are: The relapse prone ex-smoker engages in unhelpful black or white thinking. "Either I'm smoking or not, either I'm a smoker or not. So if I have one, I might as well just keep smoking." He or she exaggerates negative thoughts about self-efficacy. "I don't have any will power. I'm hopeless." Or, the "violator" uses the slip as an excuse to indulge: "I've been bad, so I might as well enjoy myself for a while before I have to get back under control."

Initial small slips usually are forced by circumstances like a sudden injury or illness. Those can snowball into a bigger lapse if the mind takes over and interprets the slips as a defect in self-control or an excuse for a holiday.

Learning new behavior doesn't mean old behavior is forgotten. The motivated exerciser hopes and assumes that his or her old bad habits are left behind. But these examples of lapses in exercise show that neither extinction nor counterconditioning destroys the original learning (wanting to relax at the sight of the couch before dinner or the great taste of chips is not forgotten), rather it (sedentary behavior or eating chips) is merely suppressed in service of the new behavior (exercise walk or healthy snacks). The old behavior is not unlearned and it can be aroused again when exposed to situations or contexts outside of those where the behavior was originally eliminated or where the new replacement behavior was learned. We also understand that just a couple exposures to the old behavior can reawaken an expectation to engage in that behavior again.

The time it takes to learn a new behavior can be much longer than the time it takes to remember the past behavior. I think a food example is something most people can relate to. Let's say you had a problem snacking too much on junk food at work. Your nice co-worker in the space next to you kept a bowl of candy on her desk for passersby to enjoy. Enjoy you did and after a while you stopped by her desk every day for some chocolate. You looked forward to it and even would think about chocolate at your desk until you finally gave in to the craving and visited the candy bowl. Then one day you went cold turkey and abruptly gave up chocolate at work and made your neighbor's desk off limit to eating. Your chocolate cravings probably were more intense at first, but after a while, maybe some weeks of being consistent and riding out the cravings, you no longer thought about eating from your neighbor's desk. Then one day in a moment of overwhelming temptation you had a chocolate slip. Maybe you felt guilty and had another. Soon you started having chocolate cravings again and making regular stops at the candy bowl.

How discouraging that all you needed was a few slips and you were back to eating off your neighbor's desk. You never forgot that behavior which is why it came back so quickly compared with how long it took to supposedly eliminate it in the beginning.

The take home message is to bounce back from a slip as soon as possible in order to avoid strengthening the old behavior. If you wait too long, you'll have to repeat the process of learning the new behavior all over again. Although it might not take as long as the first time, recovery will not be immediate. So, you should think about the consequences of slipping. If your slip turns into a relapse, you are looking forward to some hard work again.

Slips And Recovery

A slip is when you temporarily stop or skip exercise. That could involve either skipping an entire day of exercise or stopping your workout before you should have ended. It could involve skipping certain intensities or types of exercise that you should be doing. Any interruption in your exercise routine could be considered a slip, though skipping days of exercise is the most significant because frequency of exercise is the main determinant of habit strength.

A relapse is a return to your baseline, back to the way you used to be before you started a serious attempt at an exercise habit, back to zero. A slip is short lasting so you haven't lost anything really, maybe a little momentum, but basically you still want to exercise as much as before and you haven't lost any fitness. Whereas after a relapse, you've totally given up and lost the motivation and soon the fitness you had back when you were exercising regularly. A lapse is somewhere between a slip and relapse – a series of slips one after another or a break of a week or few weeks, but not such a long break from exercise that you lost hope or fitness altogether. These three types of incidents are on a continuum. A slip can lead to more slips and to a lapse and then to a relapse. Mental attitudes and beliefs confuse these three. An important step to recover from not exercising is to be realistic about how much trouble you created.

The downward cycle of slips and recovery. When you slip from your exercise habit without truly dealing with the problem, you are more likely to slip again and have more trouble recovering. A vicious cycle unfolds whereby one slip leads to another because you do not cope well enough to interrupt or prevent slipping. Pretty soon you are heading toward a lapse or relapse.

Figure 15.2 is a diagram that illustrates the downward cycle of slips over time. On the left side, the vertical axis represents the effectiveness of your exercise habit – your self-control or self-management of exercise, not your physical strength or fitness. The diagram progresses to the right, showing changes in effectiveness over time. Let's say the far left represents how strong your exercise habit or self-control was at the end of "treatment" or the end of the active phase when you achieved regular exercise.

Sometime after that point, you have a small slip, then some more slips and your exercise control reaches a low point for a while. Finally, you recover, but not back to being as strong (or as in control, confident, resilient) as before – the hump on the diagram is lower than your baseline effectiveness after "treatment". Inevitably you have another slip and because you didn't cope well, that one takes your effectiveness even lower. Notice the trough shows a longer time before you start recovering from the slip. And after you start, you do not bounce back quickly like before, rather recovery is slower this time. Then the next hump is shorter; you're in control for a shorter amount of time. After more slips, your exercise control is at a low point where it stays on hold indefinitely. This cycle usually translates into feeling out of control, discouraged and finally hopeless.

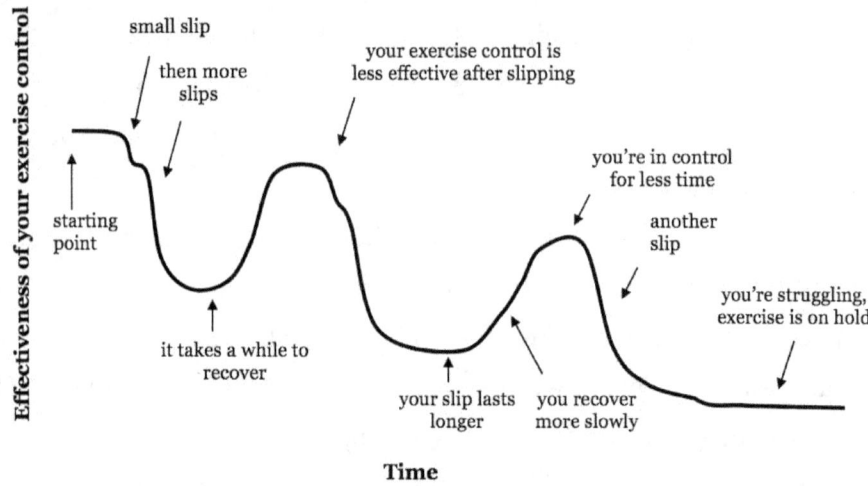

Figure 15.2 The Downward cycle of slips and recovery: poor coping with slips leads to giving-up exercise

The upward cycle of slips and recovery. The diagram of slips and recovery in Figure 15.3 is going "upward" because it is an example of how you can get better, rather than worse if you learn from the slip and practice good coping skills. This is the curve I want you to follow so you will maintain exercise.

Look at the diagram and see that after the first set of slips you took some time to recover, but you ended up being in more control of your exercise (the hump after the slip is higher than baseline). The next time you slip, the second trough on the diagram is not as low as before - you didn't slip as badly, you were less out of control; maybe you learned to prevent one slip leading to another. After recovering, you remain in good control without slipping for a longer time. Perhaps you were learning to anticipate and cope with triggers for slips. The next time you slip, the third dip in the diagram, you recovered very quickly. By this time, you are an expert at resuming your normal exercise routine making your habit stronger.

In sum, by coping well with slips you have learned more about the risk situations that trigger them, you don't slip as far, you recover more quickly, and you stay in control longer before the next slip. The downward cycle of slips shows you spend more time overall in the zone of poor exercise control. Whereas, the upward cycle of good slip management shows you spend most of your time in good and even better control than before. This is the result of repeatedly practicing good coping strategies and getting out of a slip as soon as possible.

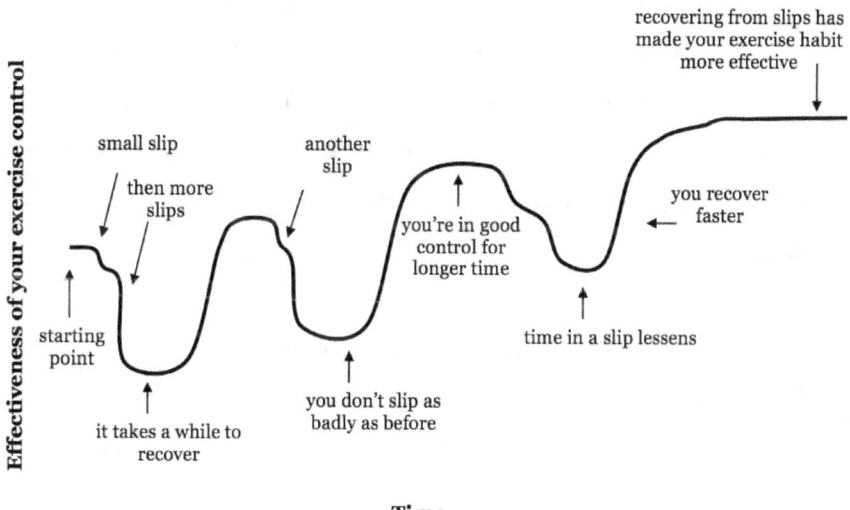

Figure 15.3 The Upward cycle of slips and recovery: good coping with slips strengthens an exercise habit

How To Cope With Slips

Certainly, slips and lapses are inevitable and learning to cope strengthens your habit. But let's be honest about the challenge ahead. To truly recover from an interruption of your exercise habit you must go through the process of exercising consistently again and although it might not take as long as the first time, recovery will not be immediate. So, you should think about the consequences of slipping. If you lapse, you are looking forward to some hard work again.

Having said that, the best way to cope with a slip is to expect it and prepare a strategy to resist or recover quickly. So, we will begin with a worksheet for you to identify your high-risk situations for slips. After I will present basic strategies to manage slips.

What are your risk situations for exercise slips? This simple questionnaire should start you thinking about triggers for slipping from exercise. You do not need to know what "caused" your slip. It's difficult to prove what causes behavior. Just focus on the circumstances. What was happening at the time? What led to what? What was going on outside or inside of you? Give your answers before reading further.

My Risk Situations For Slips

1. The last time you exercised regularly and stopped or cut back, what were the circumstances? Answer for the time before last as well.

---

2. The last time you skipped a planned exercise episode, what was happening? Answer for some skips before the last time as well.

3. What do you anticipate happening in the next few months that might make it hard to be consistent with exercise? Write as many possible interferences or triggers for not exercising as possible.

Figure 15.4 Identify situations that put you at risk for exercise slips

Check your work in previous chapters for other situations and attitudes that trigger exercise slips. Chapter 7 on self-talk helped you identify things you say to yourself that discourage exercise. Check the self-talk diary you kept and Figure 7.1 for examples. Chapter 8 on Cue Your Exercise explained that cues or stimuli could trigger exercise avoidance. Check Figure 8.2 where you might have recorded some of yours. Chapter 9 on social support discussed unsupportive people. You were to have written things that family, friends or workmates do that are not helpful. Finally, Chapter 14 about health beliefs discussed how people form thoughts about the "barriers" or disadvantages of engaging in a health behavior. Check the examples of common barriers and any you might have included in Figure 14.1, Self-talk about my health.

Are you able to identify any risks? Is there a pattern? Or do your slips seem totally random? Were your triggers something outside of you like the weather or were they inside like being in a bad mood? Do your risk situations have to do with other people? With work schedule? With holidays or change of seasons?

After you finish writing, check this partial list of common triggers for exercise slips or lapses. These might stir your thoughts about other situations that belong on your list.

Common Risks For Exercise Slips

1. travelling, away from home
2. holiday
3. too busy, time crunch, time conflict
4. sick
5. injured
6. injury, illness, death or other problem with a loved one
7. bad weather
8. bad mood
9. no exercise partner
10. people telling you not to exercise
11. change of season
12. change to standard time and less daylight
13. weight gain
14. feel bad about physical appearance
15. problems with exercise gear or equipment

Prepare for slips. If you already know your risk situations for skipping exercise, you might be able to prevent or at least interrupt slips by planning ahead. Having a plan before encountering the risky situation will make you feel in control rather than taken by surprise. The two basic steps are problem solving and rehearsal.

Problem solve. To problem solve, you state the upcoming risk situation, the different coping strategies that fit the situation, the advantages and disadvantages of each and the best of those alternatives. You have learned many behavioral and cognitive strategies to make yourself exercise. Use those to cope with a challenging situation. Following (Figure 15.5) is an example problem solving worksheet for a couple upcoming risks for slipping on exercise.

Risk for exercise slip	Possible solutions	Advantages & disadvantages	Best solution
It's supposed to start snowing tomorrow for the rest of the week. I won't be able to ride my bike.	1. Go for a long ride today before it snows	1. I don't have time to ride today	Work out in the fitness center this week
	2. Work out in the fitness center this week	2. Cardio workouts in the fitness center are boring. But this would help me to focus on weight training	
			Cont'd

Risk for exercise slip	Possible solutions	Advantages & disadvantages	Best solution
	3. Ride anyway when the roads are plowed. Wear my new weather proof riding outfit	3. I don't mind the weather but I'm worried about the bike slipping near cars	
	4. Skip exercise until the weather improves	4. This would be easy, but I'd feel guilty & out of shape not exercising so long	
The family holiday is coming. I'm concerned about eating and sitting around and missing my long Saturday walk. People won't like me taking off to exercise.	1. Walk early & arrive at the family late	1. Arriving late will hurt people's feelings	A short walk before dinner with whoever wants to join me. Positive self-talk to enjoy myself.
	2. Invite the family to take a walk with me	2. Most wouldn't be interested, but a couple people might take a short walk before dinner.	
	3. Don't eat much so I won't feel guilty	3. Not realistic. The family celebration is too yummy.	

Risk for exercise slip	Possible solutions	Advantages & disadvantages	Best solution
	4. Tell myself family is important and it's OK as long as I get a good workout the next day	4. A promise to make up for it & concentrating on family will help me not feel guilty & enjoy myself	

Figure 15.5 Worksheet to brain storm the best solution to risks for exercise slips.

Make your own problem solving worksheet now with one or more of your upcoming risks for exercise slips. Maybe you feel confident you can handle it, but don't bypass this step. Go through the motion of problem solving in writing. Written statements especially intentions to act a certain way are more effective than just thinking about it. When you prove that you can problem solve and prevent slips, it will be fine to work out solutions in your head.

Rehearse. To rehearse means you prepare yourself to encounter a risk for slipping by imagining how you might feel and how you will act. A rehearsal is more than thinking, "Oh, yeah, I'll just go to the fitness center when it starts snowing." Rehearsal means to vividly picture yourself in the situation and play through the steps you will take, like you are watching a movie.

Let's use the above examples. I close my eyes and rehearse by thinking: "It's going to snow tomorrow. I will feel grumpy about the weather and will start thinking 'there is no point to doing anything if I can't ride.' But I must go to the fitness center even though the cardio workout there is wimpy compared to riding. At least I can weight train. I need to work out with weights and am looking forward to it. I picture myself dressed in my gym clothes walking into the fitness center. I'm going to have a positive attitude."

In the family situation, I could rehearse inviting willing people to join me for a walk. It would be unusual for the family to do anything active at this occasion and people might think I'm silly. Knowing their reaction, I should picture myself acting convincing before facing them for real.

In sum, brain storm different ways to handle a risky situation. Make a mental picture of you resisting temptation to slip and performing the best solution. Repeat the image until you have it perfect. After rehearsing the solution the first time, be sure to prepare yourself right before encountering the actual risk situation. The less confident you are, the more practice you need.

Avoid risk situations. It is admirable to charge ahead and conquer exercise-killing situations, but avoidance is a perfectly legitimate coping strategy as well. Think about risk situations you identified in the previous section and cues that trigger exercise slips from the worksheet in Chapter 8 (Figure 8.2). Can you reduce your risk for slipping by simply avoiding any of these situations?

Earlier I gave the example of me trying to leave my office for a bike ride before getting involved with work or other people. It turned out that just the sight of colleagues or unfinished work on my desk was enough to distract me. Through trial and error, I learned that I needed to drop off my stuff and leave on my bike without entering the building. Or how about the classic problem of trying to exercise after getting home from work when the family wants your attention? I had clients who learned to delay exposing themselves to that exercise killer by exercising on the way home. This technique is referred to as "stimulus control" or "cue control". You are controlling by eliminating or delaying cues that trigger not exercising.

These examples are daily or minor situations. How about less frequent, but more costly risks for slipping, the kind that might turn from a slip to an extended lapse. I had a client who would vacation by chartering a private sailboat to roam around the Caribbean for a couple weeks every winter. Her problem was working fitness into being on a small boat day after day. By the time she returned home, her momentum to exercise was gone. As much as she loved sailing, she became serious about staying fit and switched to more active vacations; trips where she could hike, bike, and kayak.

Maybe there are holiday traditions, events, clubs, committees, or other pastimes that could be revised or avoided altogether in order to eliminate interferences in your schedule of regular and hopefully almost daily exercise. This reminds me of my earlier remarks on letting go of activities that might be enjoyable but must be a lower priority if you are serious about becoming physically fit. Some sacrifice must be made to achieve a healthy lifestyle.

Face risk situations. Some situations cannot or should not be avoided. Cold or nasty weather is unavoidable if you exercise outdoors. Messing your hair, even after your weekly styling might be unavoidable if you want to exercise every day. Not having your regular aerobics class on family vacations is not an acceptable excuse to skip exercise altogether. It would be self-defeating to skip your workout because you felt fat in your exercise clothes. These are situations that should be faced and overcome. Avoidance offers short-term relief from anxiety and discomfort, but prevents you from learning how to cope with the situation.

The opposite is to be hardy, to withstand adverse conditions (Chapter 11). That involves facing difficult exercise situations in order to learn solutions and to not be so bothered. Could you intentionally do your outside exercise on the nastiest of weather days just to prove you can do it and not pass on a day of exercise? Could you go ahead with your aerobics class even on a day when you think you're looking fat just to feel proud you did it? Risk situations for slips present an opportunity for "planned hardiness", times when you go out of your way to strengthen yourself by facing adversity.

The coping strategies of avoidance and facing or exposing oneself to adversity require self-control and practice. Neither type of response is better than the other. It's up to you to decide which fits the situation best and which will make your exercise habit stronger.

Use helpful self-talk. Some situations literally force you off exercise and there is nothing you could have done to prevent it. Think injury, illness. How about stressful events when exercise can't be the usual priority: a major work crunch, problem in the family or death of a loved one. Your interpretation of these slips can make the difference between a short or long break in exercise.

Some guilt or disappointment is realistic whether your slip was caused by you or was out of your control. But exaggerated negative thinking could result in an Abstinence Violation Effect. Remember, this is a paradoxical reaction whereby one needlessly concludes that to maintain exercise is hopeless after an initial minor slip. Subsequently the slip can turn into a binge on sedentary behavior if not a full-blown relapse.

The solution is to work on your rational self-talk. These are statements that correct self-defeating or false thinking by responding with a more correct or logical self-statement. Check the following table (Figure 15.6) for examples of problematic and alternative thinking after slips. Refer to Chapter 7 for tips on making self-talk more helpful.

Type Of Problem Thinking	Example	Alternative Thought
All or nothing thinking	"This is just like before. Barely a few months have gone by and I am thinking of excuses to not exercise. I'm hopeless. I don't have any willpower."	"I slipped a couple times but actually I'm exercising most of the time. I should worry but not feel hopeless. All I need to do is exercise tomorrow and not give-up."
Overgeneralizing	"I missed one aerobics class. I'll never be able to keep up with this schedule."	"I missed a class because I had a time conflict. I can make class most other times."
		Cont'd

Type Of Problem Thinking	Example	Alternative Thought
Discounting the positive	"I was walking consistently for three months, but that's only because my friend was making me. How will I do this by myself?"	"Three months is a long time for me to keep up exercise. I might not have my walking partner, but my partner wasn't the only reason I walked; I can do it on my own."
Jumping to conclusions	"I can't walk today because my knee hurts. I must have ruined my knee by walking so much. This is the end of my fitness."	"It's too soon to know what's wrong with my knee. I should stay away from walking for a while and do something else like weight train and swim."

Type Of Problem Thinking	Example	Alternative Thought
Reading people's minds	"My wife will worry that I didn't exercise on the business trip. She'll think I'm a loser. When it feels like she is nagging me, I feel like rebelling and waiting even longer to get going."	"Maybe I should ask what she thinks instead of assuming she disapproves. I think she'll understand. Anyway, I need to focus on me and start exercising again rather than make this a power struggle."
Future guessing	"Not working out this week means I won't be able to hike fast enough to keep up with my friends. Maybe I should skip the hike too."	"I can't predict what will happen at the next hike. I'll probably do fine, maybe a little slower but that doesn't mean I should skip hiking altogether."
Magnify	"I haven't exercised lately. I'm completely out of shape. Why bother starting tomorrow. I might as well wait until I feel like it."	"I'm much more fit than before. Any fitness I lost recently I can regain in a short while. The sooner I start, the better."

Figure 15.6 Be careful of overly negative thinking after exercise slips.

Positive self-talk does not need to be overly positive, just more realistic and helpful than the irrational or distorted thinking that could worsen your slip from exercise. It's okay to not believe an alternative thought 100 percent. Simply repeat your more rational talk until your slip feels under control.

Step back from your self-talk for a moment and ask why your thoughts are so negative. Do they merely reflect disappointment? Or might you subconsciously be talking that way to justify an even longer break from exercise – "I'm hopeless" is an excuse to take more time off. Or might you be trying to punish yourself – "I failed so I deserve to feel worse by letting myself get out of shape again." Positive self-talk alone will not combat hidden desires to fail. Be honest and create self-talk that fits the situation.

Reframe your slip. To reframe is technique of cognitive modification to find an alternative way of viewing a situation, like to reframe a picture with a different border or to view a scene through a different lens. More than just positive self-talk, to reframe a slip or lapse means to look at it completely differently – usually from the opposite view where you can enjoy or at least accept it graciously rather than dread it.

If you are stuck thinking, "I failed." Try reframing by focusing on an accomplishment – yes, an accomplishment: "I learned something about my risk situations for slipping. I learned I would have to be better prepared next time." Think of this as an opportunity to prove how strong and able you are to resist letting your slips snowball into bigger problem. If you didn't make mistakes or take time off from exercise, you couldn't become a slip-master.

If you are overly discouraged about losing fitness after an exercise lapse, if you are preoccupied with how hard it feels to work out now, reframe that by anticipating your fitness improving again. At the beginning you probably felt excited about the results of starting to exercise more. If after a lapse, it's like starting all over again, you probably will progress quickly and return to where you left off. Enjoy the opportunity, because after it's an easy routine again, it won't be as exciting.

If you are bummed about gaining weight from not exercising, reframe the situation as one you have control over – you can lower your weight again like before. Weigh yourself – don't avoid it – and watch the number on the scale go down. Feel in control, rather than out of control.

Refresh your health beliefs. The initiation of a new health behavior like exercise is more likely if you believe it will benefit your health and prevent disease. These are beliefs about outcomes in the future. After changing the behavior, if you are satisfied with the outcome you are likely to think you made the right decision and to continue the behavior.

I knew someone who was working hard to improve his fitness. When I asked if he did any cardio work in addition to his regular strength training, he said, "Oh, I tried that, I was running everyday but stopped. It didn't do anything for me." Surprised, I asked what he meant by it not doing anything. He said, "I didn't feel any better, any more fit." I asked what changes he did notice and he replied that it took less time to run the same distance and admitted he must have been running faster. I said, "Well, running faster is better fitness. Your running was working." Clearly, this fellow gave-up because he expected something more than ordinary aerobic conditioning.

In the field of weight control, to lose ten percent of body weight is usually associated with significant improvements in physical health.

For many obese persons, that is enough to reduce or stop medication and to function better in daily life. Yet if you ask people who weigh 250 pounds before they start a weight loss program, "Would you be happy if you lost 25 pounds" the answer is usually, "No". Not surprising. If one reduces to 225 pounds (loses ten percent), he or she still would be obese and certainly not the thin image the person might have hoped for. Fortunately, the human psyche has a way of adjusting to circumstances. Most end-up being satisfied with a weight loss that at the beginning they predicted would be a failure. That is because they feel better and are healthier and they recognize what they accomplished. Incidentally, a benchmark of success in weight control is ten percent weight loss. Achieving that in and of itself is something to be proud of since most people in weight control programs do not.

The next time you struggle with overcoming exercise slips, when you feel ambivalent about persevering and think it isn't worth it, stop and review the benefits you expected (Figure 14.2). Think about what you have accomplished. If less than expected, are your accomplishments desirable nonetheless? Can you find some satisfaction in exercising that makes it worth continuing? Can you revise your expectations and bring them in line better with the actual results? Shift your thinking from this isn't worthwhile to why it is.

Restart from the beginning. If you regressed so badly that you feel overwhelmed, no worry, start doing the basic things that made you exercise in the beginning. The first step is to start self-monitoring again and keep an exercise diary. Just like before, write your exercise information for every day. Write zero if you did nothing. Recording days of no exercise is as important as exercise days. Remember, the point is more than to have data on yourself, it's to motivate you to increase the desirable behavior. It's normal to want to avoid looking at yourself if you feel you are doing badly, but avoidance prolongs getting behavior under control. Studies of successful weight losers show that the first action they take when starting to slip is to resume an eating diary.

The second step in making yourself exercise is to increase exercise frequency. If you have lapsed and feel discouraged, do not worry about returning to the same routine immediately. Lower your expectations. Simply start by doing something on one day, then the next day and so on until you are doing some amount of physical activity most days. Do not worry about the amount of time or quality of exercise. Simply go through the motions of restarting exercise behavior and let the techniques you learned do their magic. It won't be long before you return to where you left off.

Take action quickly. A few slips are enough to reinstate old behavior that really hasn't been forgotten and still lurks beneath the surface. You prevent long lapses or relapse by keeping the recovery time from a slip to a minimum. What matters is not how long you continuously exercise, rather the quickness with which you recover from taking a break. Do not procrastinate.

It's hard to get back into exercise after a week, two weeks or more time off. Make yourself do something as soon as possible even if it's less than your normal workout, simply to prove you are still an exerciser and to restart your momentum. If you exercise today, the probability of exercise tomorrow is greater. It's that simple. Past behavior predicts future behavior. Look again at Figure 15.3 and think of slips as having a shape or pattern over time. Two features are the length of time in between slips and the length of time to recover from slips. In that example of the "Upward cycle" or good coping, these features improve. Make a conscious commitment to recover more quickly than last time. Speedy recovery is a skill that takes practice.

Cope with holidays and travel. To these we can add other typical risk situations for slips including bad weather, injury, illness and weight gain. The risk for slipping in these circumstances is simply due to lack of practice. We tend to exercise when conditions are right, easy, convenient and so forth and do not practice exercise when we are away from home, when the weather is bad and so forth. The best solution is to develop a high frequency of exercise as recommended throughout this book. When you are doing something 6 or 7 days a week, inevitably you learn to associate exercise with many cues. Your exercise habit is stronger and you expect to exercise regardless of the situation. So, if you are having slips and generally have a low exercise frequency (4 days or less per week), after you are back in control, gradually increase your regular frequency to daily or almost daily exercise. This will boost your resistance to slipping the next time.

These high-risk situations also test a person's flexibility. Cold weather, being away from home, having an injury might prevent your favorite form of exercise, but not all forms of exercise. Having a wide repertoire of physical activity lets you pick something else that fits the situation. If you depend on aerobics classes at the fitness center, feeling comfortable with exercise walks is important if you are to be active when you're away from home. If your knee pain stops you from running, cycling or swimming can be a substitute until you're able to run again. Exercise the part of your body that is working.

Varying exercise intensity is handy for slip management. If you are in a time crunch and tempted to skip your workout altogether, why not squeeze-in a shorter high intensity or recovery workout. To vary type and intensity of exercise will improve your fitness. And from a psychological point of view, becoming less rigid and more varied will boost your resistance to slipping.

If you are totally off exercise waiting to recover from an injury, it's normal to feel a sense of loss; loss of fun, loss of fitness, loss of the habit you worked so hard to create. But avoiding harmful activity is important for physical rehabilitation. You do not have a choice. It's not your fault. Externally caused lapses are usually easier to deal with due to less self-blame. The event is not evidence for some internal defect. Stay focused on this coping attitude with appropriate self-talk. Re-frame the event as an opportunity for some positive outcome. When you're ready to re-start exercise, go back to the basics like self-monitoring and gradual increases in activity.

Get help again. If you regained weight after dieting, you might say, "that diet didn't work." But in weight control, the problem is not that dieting doesn't work – people usually lose weight - rather that people wait too long to start weight control again. Instead of stopping after losing weight, people who keep going and get structured help for a whole year end up losing more weight than people in a normal length program. Being overweight is a chronic issue and one treatment program, especially just a couple months of help, will not permanently end it for most people.

If you worked out in a fitness center and after quitting you lost muscle, you shouldn't say "that fitness center didn't work." It just means you stopped doing the exercise and might need to rejoin in order to maintain your fitness. I had a client who started her exercise habit by working with a trainer at her health club. She made an agreement with herself that if she did not keep up her routine on her own, she would immediately schedule supervised exercise again. The longer you stay in a program or the shorter you wait to start again, the better will be your exercise.

There should be no shame to getting help if you lapsed. Join an exercise class, get an exercise buddy, or work with a trainer. Sometimes a structured, formal or professional service that makes you exercise is necessary to start again. If it works, why not get outside help if you are not doing it on your own.

Are you suffering from overtraining? Sometimes a slip is not a slip, but our body telling us we need to take a break from intense exercise in order to recover physically. If you work out in the higher aerobic intensity zones almost every day, you may be in need of some easy days. Dedicated exercisers can misinterpret urges to cut back on exercise as a slip into sloth and then make the problem worse by exercising harder than they really should to prove they are still fit. Eventually, a break is forced on the over-exerciser by illness, fatigue, or loss of motivation. If your slip fits into this scenario, go back to Chapter 10 and create a healthier exercise schedule with workouts that vary intensity and recovery. Remember, recovery does not mean vegetating on the couch – that would be a slip. Recovery is being active but at a lower intensity. If what really is happening is a need to recover, take advantage of it. Enjoy some lower intensity activity.

Make yourself have a slip. This sounds strange, but how can you practice slip management if you never have one? Over the years in my weight control program, participants who resisted change and had trouble losing weight were troublesome of course. But I also worried about people who were perfect: people who stuck to the program and followed every recommendation without fail, lost weight every week, and never transgressed. Although they were doing well in the program, I worried what might happen later when they were on their own and I was not around to help them cope with a slip. Indeed, sometimes perfect people take the biggest fall when they encounter that inevitable disruption of their perfect behavior.

I challenged these perfect participants to intentionally slip by eating some food off their diet or by skipping exercise. Naturally, this triggered anxiety in my clients and that was exactly the reaction I hoped to produce. Included in the anxiety reaction might be upsetting thoughts that accompany an Abstinence Violation Effect such as: "I feel guilty", "I blew it", "I'll get out of shape", "I'll get fat". I had faith my clients would cope with the negative thoughts and feelings and recover from the slip without spiraling down. Facing a slip, albeit artificially induced, helped my clients be less worried when they faced real ones.

Yes, I'm suggesting that if you have been perfect, make yourself have a slip. The best slip would be one that exposes you to feelings of guilt, worry, and maybe temptation to keep slipping. If skipping one day isn't enough, skip a few days until you experience some distress about not exercising. The purpose is not to take an exercise rest, but to practice confronting feelings in a controlled manner that you might confront later in the middle of a crisis and when you might be more vulnerable. Think of this as an inoculation against a worse reaction when the real thing happens.

Control slips on self-management skills. Self-management skills are the behaviors that helped you to start and to continue exercising. Self-monitoring, positive self-talk, cue control, assertiveness with other people, prioritizing exercise, self-reward and so forth are behaviors that lead up to exercising. You should be as worried about letting go of those behaviors as letting go of exercise itself. If you start having trouble maintaining your exercise routine, review the self-management chapters and the techniques you used earlier that helped you develop an exercise habit. Reestablish those behaviors and hopefully you will find it easier to prevent more slips.

Remember that returning to basic strategies like keeping an exercise record is one of the best ways to motivate yourself.

Focus on a different health behavior. Health behaviors tend to correlate with one another, which means they influence each other or share a common influence. As a result, changing one behavior can lead to improvement in another behavior that was not targeted.

My last resort recommendation to people who are failing to exercise is to find a different health behavior to change. The hope is that working on something else will trigger improvement in exercise. Having a primary care provider is a health behavior, but it's hard to imagine that acquiring one would cause a person to start exercising. Drug and alcohol use, overeating and poor nutrition, and smoking are health risks that could make exercise more difficult and seem more logically connected. So, working on one of those would be a good choice.

Here is an example of this concept from my weight control program. Some people have great trouble eating less food and the more pressure they feel, the more out of control they become. It's as if food, eating, and weight have all kinds of psychological overtones and the person is stuck in a conflict between self-indulgence and self-denial. My recommendation was to put the diet part of the program on hold and simply work on increasing exercise. Exercise does not have as much psychological baggage as food and might be easier to control. For some people, adding a behavior (exercise) is easier than taking away a behavior (eating). After some success with exercise, diet could be addressed once more.

Let's consider an exercise example. Cigarette smoking impairs cardiorespiratory functioning and can make it harder and less pleasant to exercise. Which behavior should be targeted first? One could make a case for either or both simultaneously, but if you personally absolutely cannot make yourself exercise, maybe switching to the smoking problem might be better. It certainly makes sense that quitting smoking might make exercise feel less bad. And maybe you are the type of person who does better with an all-or-nothing change like quitting smoking.

There is no point to feeling like a failure on an ongoing basis. Pick the behavior you can control now.

Transition To Maintenance

We are reaching the conclusion of this guide to create an exercise habit. And as we do, hopefully you are past the point of learning new behavior and are ready to maintain your habit. Maintenance is after the education phase. It's when supposedly you are ready to keep what you accomplished and to continue change on your own. This is a time to be proud and perhaps a little anxious. After all, you probably have been in this situation before when you thought you solved your exercise problem and later you had to read this book to solve it again. I recommend you reflect on your feelings and thoughts about this transition. Answer the following questions to guide your next steps toward creating a lasting exercise habit.

What is My Attitude About Maintaining Exercise?

1. How confident are you about your accomplishments? How strong is your exercise habit (reassess yourself with the questionnaire in Figure 4.1)? Are you looking forward to working on your own without structured help like this book? In what way are your feelings mixed?

2. Have you gone as far with your fitness as you want or need to? In what ways, yes and in what ways, no?

3. Are you looking to the near future as a time to take a break from being disciplined about exercise or do you see yourself working hard?

4. Do you remember and understand why you didn't exercise enough and got out of shape before this program? How can you use this understanding to prevent a relapse in the future?

5. To what extent did you start exercising in order to prove something to someone else? Have you internalized the need for exercise and good fitness, that is, made the changes for yourself?

6. Sometimes other people act like you are over your problem because you're exercising and in better shape, when in fact you feel like you're still struggling. What reactions are you getting? In what way do they help or not help?

7. People read books like this for extra support and motivation. Maybe you also had other people who supported you. Do you have a way to stay committed on your own? Do you have a way to hold yourself accountable?

8. People can be reluctant to admit a desire for further help. You may think you can manage satisfactorily on your own. Or you may feel a need for continuing assistance. What is your attitude about receiving more help?

9. Do you have a goal that is motivating you to keep going with your exercise (for example: lose weight, become more fit, perform a sport better, get off medication)?

10. Have you been working to your best ability? Do you try new challenges to improve your exercise? Are you consistent in following good self-management strategies? Are you honest with yourself about your fitness effort? Why or why not?

Figure 15.7 Reflect on the transition from the education to maintenance phase.

Which of these questions do you relate to the most? What have you learned about yourself and what should you do to address any concerns?

Conclusion

The maintenance of new, positive health behavior is complex. I tried to remove some of the mystery by presenting information on the factors that cause people to have lapses in their exercise and how to recover from them. Regardless of what interruptions to exercise you may face or how you cope, the bottom line for creating a lasting habit comes to this. Do not delay. Recover from slips and lapses as soon as possible. Continue regular exercise for longer and longer intervals before having another break. Keep going, month after month to deepen your habit and reduce the risk for future interruptions.

Chapter 16:
Conclusion

Physical activity is less important in daily work today. Passive sedentary leisure is more common. And a vicious cycle has resulted whereby there is less need to exercise, fewer people are exercisers, and inactivity is accepted and even encouraged. Adding these cultural factors to the physical effort and time required for physical recreation, wanting to skip exercise is understandable. That's why I called this book, "How to Make Yourself Exercise." I wanted to give you a strategy to create the initial motivation and momentum to overcome these barriers. The two techniques most important at the beginning are to measure exercise every day and to gradually increase the frequency or number of days with exercise. It's best to be patient, keep your expectations low, and not worry about the quality of your exercise.

After this initial phase, the challenge is to make exercise more like a habit, something that is automatic and does not involve a lot of conscious effort and mental argument. That requires making exercise frequent, adaptive to circumstances, and associated with many situations. Some of the important techniques to deepen an exercise habit are to fulfill goals, to vary the type and intensity of exercise, to face fears or challenging situations, and to control excuses and negative thinking.

A new habit takes longer than just a few weeks. Thankfully, the probability of a relapse decreases the longer you stick to an exercise routine. So, very simply, the secret to "Creating a Lasting Habit" comes down to exercising regularly longer over time without a significant break. Breaks do happen, of course, and the most important response is to keep the break as short as possible. Hopefully, having slips will reveal your risk situations so you can be prepared to act more quickly next time. After months of exercising you should have a good repertoire of cognitive and behavioral strategies to cope with slips. An important one is to immediately resume self-monitoring of exercise behavior because that keeps your attention focused on it. Another is to have a constructive attitude about the slip itself. Too much guilt and worry about relapse might make you feel hopeless unnecessarily and give-up. Too little concern might allow you to procrastinate until you really do have to start all over.

Physical activity is so lacking in our lifestyle that the goal for exercise has been set really low by government public health agencies. Yes, some physical activity is better than nothing at the beginning. But after reaching an easier exercise goal, you should keep going to build the volume of activity in your lifestyle until you exercise every day or almost every day for at least six hours per week. Most bodies are capable of that. It's a matter of becoming more time efficient and letting go of other time occupying activity that does not contribute to health. Real health and fitness result from lots of time being physical. If you're serious about improving your fitness, there is no choice but to make the time for it.

Health experts often remark that if exercise came in pill form, it would be the most sought-after drug on the market. Nearly every ailment, effect of aging, and activity of daily living are improved by exercise. A lack of exercise leads to shorter life. Our human physiology today was formed long ago when our ancestors worked physically all day. Now we, the descendants do not expose ourselves to the physical demand our bodies were designed for. That's like withdrawing medicine or nourishment that our physiology came to expect. When you don't like exercise, you might have to think about it as medicine that you need to take.

The normal trend over adulthood is to allow progressively less time for physical recreation. Around the beginning of middle age is when aging and the loss of fitness become more noticeable. It's not until then that most people recognize they've been losing health and vitality. Attempts to start exercising again are most likely in the forties and procrastination usually ends when high blood pressure, high cholesterol, or overweight materializes. Sadly, when the attempt fails, people usually procrastinate another five years before trying again. Why wait for a wake-up call to your health? Do it now.

The approach you learned in this book is behavioral self-management. It uses techniques that help people to control themselves and learn new behavior. You are in charge of your behavior change; it's up to you. Either you want to exercise more or you don't. You can't have everything – add exercise and keep everything else the same. If you follow the instructions and practice, you will change. Don't cut corners. Take some risks. Try new challenges. Reach out for help. Do it for yourself because you want to not because someone or something is making you. Ask yourself, "Am I working to the best of my ability?"

And now I say goodbye and I wish you the best on changing your health behavior and becoming a regular exerciser. Enjoy.

www.ingramcontent.com/pod-product-compliance
Lightning Source LLC
Chambersburg PA
CBHW071331280526
45787CB00001B/68